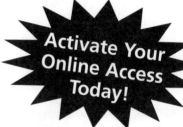

theclinics.com

ORAL AND MAXILLOFACIAL SURGERY CLINICS

of North America

Minimally Invasive Cosmetic
Facial Surgery

JOSEPH NIAMTU III, DMD
Guest Editor

RICHARD H. HAUG, DDS
Consulting Editor

February 2005 • Volume 17 • Number 1

SAUNDERS

An Imprint of Elsevier, Inc.
PHILADELPHIA LONDON TORONTO MONTREAL SYDNEY TOKYO

W.B. SAUNDERS COMPANY
A Division of Elsevier Inc.

The Curtis Center • Independence Square West • Philadelphia, Pennsylvania 19106

http://www.oralmaxsurgery.theclinics.com

ORAL AND MAXILLOFACIAL SURGERY CLINICS OF NORTH AMERICA
February 2005
Editor: John Vassallo

Volume 17, Number 1
ISBN 1-4160-2839-0

Oral and Maxillofacial Surgery Clinics of North America (ISSN 1042-3699) is published quarterly by W.B. Saunders Company. Corporate and editorial offices: The Curtis Center, Independence Square West, Philadelphia, PA 19106-3399. Accounting and circulation offices: 6277 Sea Harbor Drive, Orlando, FL 32887-4800. Periodicals postage paid at Orlando, FL 32862, and additional mailing offices. Subscription prices are $180.00 per year for US individuals, $280.00 per year for US institutions, $90.00 per year for US students and residents, $208.00 per year for Canadian individuals, $325.00 per year for Canadian institutions, $225.00 per year for international individuals, $325.00 per year for international institutions and $113.00 per year for Canadian and foreign students/residents. To receive student/resident rate, orders must be accompanied by name or affiliated institution, date of term, and the *signature* of program/residency coordinator on institution letterhead. Orders will be billed at individual rate until proof of status is received. Foreign air speed delivery is included in all *Clinics* subscription prices. All prices are subject to change without notice. POSTMASTER: Send address changes to *Oral and Maxillofacial Surgery Clinics of North America,* W.B. Saunders Company, Periodicals Fulfillment, Orlando, FL 32887-4800. **Customer Service: 1-800-654-2452 (US). From outside of the US, call 1-407-345-4000.**

Printed in the United States of America.

CONSULTING EDITOR

RICHARD H. HAUG, DDS, Professor of Oral and Maxillofacial Surgery, Executive Associate Dean, University of Kentucky College of Dentistry, Lexington, Kentucky

GUEST EDITOR

JOSEPH NIAMTU III, DMD, Oral/Maxillofacial and Cosmetic Facial Surgery, Richmond, Virginia

CONTRIBUTORS

BRUCE B. CHISHOLM, MD, DDS, Rancho Mirage, California

L. ANGELO CUZALINA, MD, DDS, Private Practice and Director, Cosmetic Surgery Fellowship, Tulsa Surgical Arts; Associate Professor, Department of Oral and Maxillofacial Surgery, University of Oklahoma, Tulsa, Oklahoma; and Associate Professor, Department of Oral and Maxillofacial Surgery, University of Alabama, Birmingham, Alabama

DESMOND FERNANDES, MB, BCh, FRCS(Edin), Plastic Surgeon, The Shirnel Clinic and Department of Plastic Reconstructive Surgery, University of Cape Town, Cape Town, Heerengracht, South Africa

JOHN FLYNN, MB, BS, Dip OBST, RACOG, FRACGP, Dip P DERM, FACCS, Fellow, Australasian College of Cosmetic Surgery; and Cosmedic Clinic, Ashmore City, Gold Coast, Australia

STEVEN B. HOPPING, MD, FACS, The Center for Cosmetic Surgery; and Clinical Professor in Surgery, George Washington University, Washington, District of Columba

MICHAEL A.C. KANE, MD, Attending Surgeon, Department of Plastic Surgery, Manhattan Eye, Ear, and Throat Hospital, New York, New York

JAMES KOEHLER, MD, DDS, Cosmetic Surgery Fellow, Tulsa Surgical Arts, Tulsa, Oklahoma; and Assistant Professor, Department of Oral and Maxillofacial Surgery, University of Alabama, Birmingham, Alabama

JOSEPH NIAMTU III, DMD, Oral/Maxillofacial and Cosmetic Facial Surgery, Richmond, Virginia

SUZAN OBAGI, MD, Director, Cosmetic Surgery and Skin Health Center; and Assistant Professor of Dermatology, University of Pittsburgh Medical Center, Pittsburgh, Pennsylvania

CRAIG E. VIGLIANTE, DMD, MD, Group Private Practice, Midlothian, Virginia

CONTENTS

FORTHCOMING ISSUES

May 2005

Diagnosis and Management of Skin Cancer
Michael S. Goldwasser, DDS, MD and
Jonathan S. Bailey, DMD, MD, *Guest Editors*

August 2005

The Role of the OMS in Emergencies, Disasters, and Terrorist Attacks
Lt. Col. David B. Powers, DMD, MD, *Guest Editor*

PREVIOUS ISSUES

November 2004

Update in Craniofacial Surgery
Ramon L. Ruiz, DMD, MD, *Guest Editor*

August 2004

Odontogenic Tumors
Dean K. White, DDS, MSD, *Guest Editor*

May 2004

Lasers in Oral and Maxillofacial Surgery
Robert A. Strauss, DDS, MD and
Steven A. Guttenberg, DDS, MD, *Guest Editors*

ELSEVIER
SAUNDERS

Oral Maxillofacial Surg Clin N Am 17 (2005) ix – x

ORAL AND MAXILLOFACIAL SURGERY CLINICS of North America

Foreword

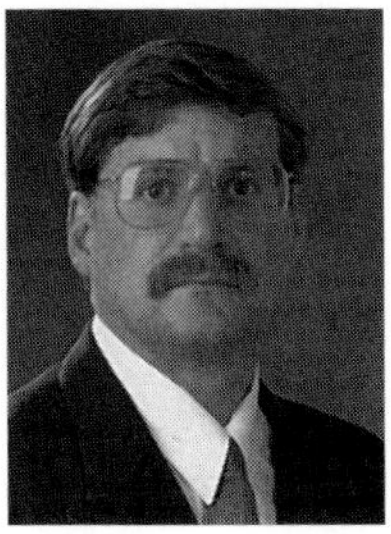

Richard H. Haug, DDS
Consulting Editor

It is with a great deal of enthusiasm and excitement that I approach serving as the new Consulting Editor for the *Oral and Maxillofacial Surgery Clinics of North America*. The *Clinics* have served Oral and Maxillofacial Surgery and related specialties for more than a decade and a half. The series has acted as a unique educational resource, complementing the cutting edge research provided in the *Journal of Oral and Maxillofacial Surgery* by relating state-of-the-art management of surgical problems in a "how to do it" fashion. Although the topics reviewed have been timely, the layout and design elegant, and the attention to detail flawless, we now have unique opportunities to refine the *Clinics*, with a different focus on the delivery of this educational product along with greater coordination with its sister publication, the *Atlas of the Oral and Maxillofacial Surgery Clinics of North America.*

Whereas the *Atlas* has striven to be a highly visual operative guide, the *Clinics* remain as an authoritative treatise on a particular subject. Over the years, we hope to provide *Clinics* and *Atlas* issues that complement each other. We will also attempt to provide summary issues of focused scientific meetings or seminars and occasional point/counter-point issues. The topics will remain focused on what is at the forefront of our specialty regarding new ideas and technology but will also provide updates of the traditional scope of practice by opinion leaders in their particular field of expertise. I hope that readers will share my enthusiasm and excitement by providing suggestions and feedback to make the next decade and a half of the *Clinics* as successful as the last.

Cosmetic Oral and Maxillofacial Surgery has become one of the eleven core clinical areas of interest in Oral and Maxillofacial Surgery, due in no small part to the contributions of surgeons like Dr. Joseph Niamtu. Dr. Niamtu has been steadfast in his commitment to our specialty, tireless in his devotion to its advancement, and unyielding in its defense. Dr. Niamtu's dedication continues with this volume devoted to Minimally Invasive Cosmetic Facial Surgery. He has coordinated the efforts of numerous experts in the field of Cosmetic Oral and Maxillofacial Surgery, each with his or her own subspecialty interest and expertise. The result is a state-of-the-art update that is thorough, detailed, easy to read, and comprehensive. Some of the topics that have been included are Botox injections for facial rejuvenation, new lip and wrinkle fillers, submentoplasty and facial liposuction, facial augmentation and volume restoration, and minimally invasive percutaneous collagen induction, to name a few. This comprehensive compendium complements the recent

1042-3699/05/$ – see front matter
doi:10.1016/j.coms.2004.10.003

two-part *Atlas of the Oral and Maxillofacial Surgery Clinics of North America* coordinated by Dr. John Griffin. Although the present issue contains different authors and subjects, the combined series reflect the collective efforts of some of our specialties' brightest rising stars.

Richard H. Haug, DDS
Professor of Oral and Maxillofacial Surgery
Executive Associate Dean
University of Kentucky College of Dentistry
Lexington, KY 40536-0297, USA
E-mail address: rhhaug2@uky.edu

ELSEVIER
SAUNDERS

Oral Maxillofacial Surg Clin N Am 17 (2005) xi – xii

ORAL AND MAXILLOFACIAL SURGERY CLINICS of North America

Preface

Minimally Invasive Cosmetic Facial Surgery

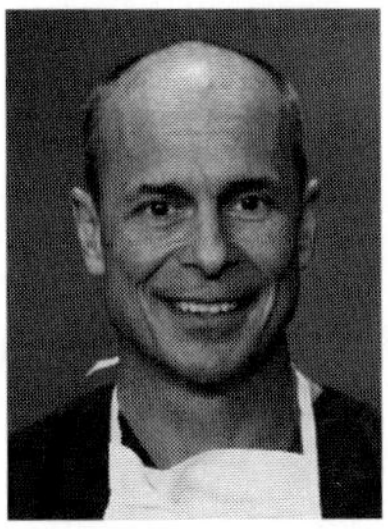

Joseph Niamtu III, DMD
Guest Editor

It is my distinct honor to have been asked to guest edit another issue of the *Oral and Maxillofacial Surgery Clinics of North America*. In November 2000, I had the honor to edit an issue on Cosmetic Facial Surgery. That volume is certainly a keeper due to the variety of contributing authors and serves as an excellent primer on cosmetic surgery techniques such as skin care, eyelid surgery, and Botox. I am told by the publisher that the 2000 issue remains a highly requested reprint. I am confident that this current issue on Minimally Invasive Cosmetic Facial Surgery will also remain a favorite, again because of the reputation of the contributing authors and their quality of work.

In the four short years since the 2000 edition, much has changed in the field of cosmetic facial surgery. There are techniques that are common now (Intense Pulsed Light (IPL), Restylane, Advanta facial implants) that were not even available in 2000, which is testament to the fast rate of change and innovation in cosmetic surgery.

With the baby boomers entering their fifth decade, there is no shortage of cosmetic patients. Cosmetic surgery is more popular than ever. This popularity is also underlined by the emergence of cosmetic surgery reality television shows. Cosmetic surgery is a hot topic in our society. Like all disciplines, the public has extreme interest for "what is hot and what is not." The populous is especially interested in procedures that are new, have short or no recovery time, and produce a noticeable difference. To that end, this text should be a valuable addition for those doctors who have an interest in cosmetic facial surgery.

Readers of this series will notice that there has been a significant increase in cosmetic surgery topics in the *Oral and Maxillofacial Surgery Clinics of North America* and the *Atlas of the Oral and Maxillofacial Surgery Clinics of North America*. This increase is representative of the role of the profession of oral and maxillofacial surgery in cosmetic facial surgery. Although there are competing professions that for reasons of turf and economics attempt to dissuade the public with inaccuracies about the role of our profession in cosmetic facial surgery, cosmetic facial surgery is one of the fastest growing aspects of our profession.

It is my hope that this text will serve to bring light to cosmetic facial surgery in our profession and serve as a reference and a guide to what I believe are exciting procedures. I am proud to have assembled such an authoritative list of contributing authors from a diverse group of specialties that deal with cosmetic surgery. In addition, the rise in the popularity of any procedure will spark a similar rise in the legal profession with lawsuits concerning these procedures. Attorney Scott Johnson is an authority on defending doctors—including oral and maxillofacial surgeons—and his input on how to protect our practices and

1042-3699/05/$ – see front matter
doi:10.1016/j.coms.2004.10.005

patients is welcomed. Dr. Des Fernandes is a plastic surgeon and recognized speaker from South Africa who is one of the most forward-thinking cosmetic surgeons I have ever had the opportunity to meet and hear. He describes a truly minimally invasive means of facial resurfacing that is innovative. Michael Kane is a renowned plastic surgeon who is an international authority on Botox. His input on Botox usage in the lower face is quite innovative. I personally caution every surgeon: these Botox techniques in the lower face are not for the novice injector and should be attempted by only those doctors with significant experience with Botox in the upper face. I have included input from Dr. Steve Hopping from ENT/ Facial Plastics who discusses the S-Lift and input from the famous dermatologist Dr. Suzan Obagi. Dr. Obagi is an ardent supporter of our profession and is one of the brightest up-and-coming stars in the field of cosmetic facial surgery. Dr. John Flynn provides some excellent input on the international status of cosmetic procedures and represents the Australasian experience. Drs. Angelo Cuzalina, James Koehler, and Bruce Chisholm truly are innovators in our profession and their command of cosmetic facial surgery has always impressed me. My associate Dr. Craig Vigliante and I have also attempted to provide useful information on facial anatomy and new procedures, respectively.

I hope that readers will learn as much from reading this issue as I learned from editing it.

Joseph Niamtu III, DMD
Oral/Maxillofacial and Cosmetic Facial Surgery
10230 Cherokee Road
Richmond, VA 23235, USA
E-mail address: niamtu@niamtu.com

ELSEVIER
SAUNDERS

Oral Maxillofacial Surg Clin N Am 17 (2005) 1 – 15

ORAL AND MAXILLOFACIAL SURGERY CLINICS of North America

Anatomy and Functions of the Muscles of Facial Expression

Craig E. Vigliante, DMD, MD

Group Private Practice, 11319 Polo Place, Midlothian, VA 23113, USA

Oral and maxillofacial surgeons have an intimate connection with the anatomy of the head and neck due to our educational background and the large amount of time spent operating in this area on a daily basis. The high degree of complexity and intricate detail of the anatomy of the facial region should be respected by even the most competent surgeons. The oral and maxillofacial surgeon's "love affair" with facial anatomy makes our profession fun and challenging.

The twenty-first century has revealed an explosion in the public's craving for cosmetic surgery. The baby-boomer generation has grasped this craze wholeheartedly. Everyone seems to be searching for the "fountain of youth." The media has been instrumental in fueling this renaissance, with television shows such as "Extreme Makeover," and "The Swan." CNN also has taken a "time-out" from its typical news coverage to expose the yearning desire of the aging population to feel young again. As surgeons of the head and neck, we are living in an age where the demand for cosmetic surgery is very high. Regardless of the surgical specialty, patients will be coming into our offices asking questions about state-of-the-art products or procedures that they have seen on television. It is our job to inform them appropriately. We need to acquire the knowledge base to provide these products or procedures. Essential to this knowledge base is a complete understanding of facial anatomy and its response to any given intervention.

The "muscles of facial expression" are manipulated by cosmetic facial surgeons to camouflage the aging process. Interventions to these muscles have profound effects on the upper, middle, and lower thirds of the face. Muscular facial activity and its relationship to the formation of wrinkles is one of the major forces responsible for facial aging. Dividing the face into muscular thirds will define the muscular groups responsible for the formation of the lines, creases, furrows, and folds that are so indicative of the aging process.

The facial musculature

The muscles of facial expression are the "cosmetic muscles." They are responsible for hyperdynamic facial lines associated with aging. These muscles have some common characteristics. They are very superficial and originate from the bones or fascia of the face. They insert into or have an influence on the skin or mucous membrane. They are second branchial arch derivatives and are supplied by the seventh cranial nerve (facial nerve). There are 40 muscles of facial expression. These muscles include the frontal bellies of the occipitofrontalis (also known as frontalis), corrugator supercilii, procerus (also known as pyramidalis nasi), orbicularis oculi, levator labii superioris alaeque nasi, nasalis, levator labii superioris, zygomaticus major, zygomaticus minor, auricularis anterior, auricularis superior, auricularis posterior, risorius, depressor septi, levator anguli oris, orbicularis oris, depressor labii inferioris, men-

The author was formerly the Chief Resident in the Department of Oral and Maxillofacial Surgery at the University of Pennsylvania Medical Center, Philadelphia, Pennsylvania.

E-mail address: vigliante@oralfacialsurgery.com

doi:10.1016/j.coms.2004.09.005

oralmaxsurgery.theclinics.com

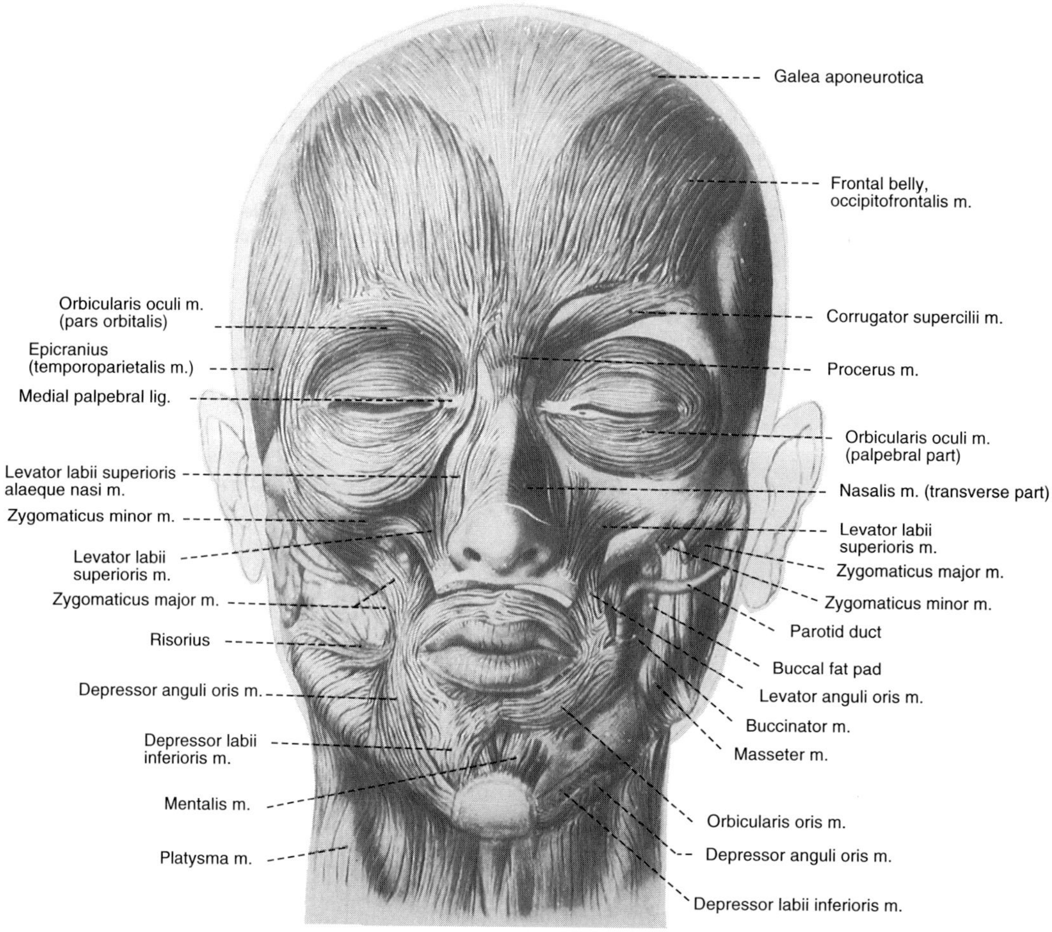

Fig. 1. The facial muscles, anterior view. On the right (reader's left) is shown the more superficial layer, whereas on the left are the deeper muscles. (*From* Putz R, Pabst R. Atlas der anatomie des menschen. 21st edition. p. 444, copyright 2000, Elsevier GmbH, Urban and Fischer Verlag Munchen; with permission.)

talis, buccinator, depressor anguli oris, and platysma (Fig. 1). Anatomically, the levator palpebrae superioris muscle is classified as an extraocular eye muscle because it is supplied by cranial nerve III; therefore, it is not grouped with the muscles of facial expression. This muscle is discussed in this article, however, because it is a direct antagonist of the orbicularis oculi muscle and a significant landmark during cosmetic surgery of the eyelids.

These muscles can be subdivided further into six groups according to their location on the head. The groups include the scalp or epicranium, the extrinsic muscles of the ear, and the muscles of the eyelids, nose, mouth, and neck. Within these muscle groups, the individual muscles can be cosmetically categorized as facial elevators and facial depressors. The anatomic review of these muscles in relation to cosmetic surgical techniques is discussed because their treatment causes physical changes in the upper, middle, and lower thirds of the face.

The musculature of the upper facial third

This group of muscles can be defined by their action on the forehead, brow, and eyes. They include the muscles of the scalp and muscles of the eyelids. These muscles include the frontalis, procerus, corrugator supercilii, orbicularis oculi, and levator palpebrae superioris (Fig. 2). Some of these muscles act as elevators and others act as depressors. Each of these

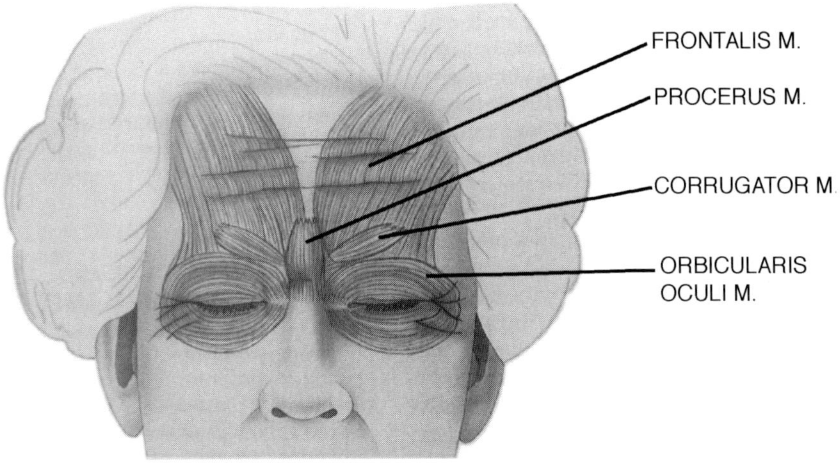

Fig. 2. Hyperdynamic facial lines, crow's feet, and glabelar furrows from activation of the muscles of the upper facial third. (*From* Zimbler MS, Kokoska MS, Thomas JR. Anatomy and pathophysiology of facial aging. Facial Plast Surg Clin N Am 2001;9(2):184; with permission.)

muscles is described in detail along with its relevance to cosmetic facial surgery.

The frontalis muscle (elevator of the brow)

This muscle is part of a larger muscle called the occipitofrontalis, which consists of two occipital bellies posteriorly, two frontal bellies anteriorly, and the galea aponeurotica (also known as epicranial aponeurosis) in between. The two frontal bellies (frontalis) and the galea aponeurotica are the anatomic parts of the occipitofrontalis that are important landmarks for cosmetic facial surgery. The occipitalis muscle is not dissected during cosmetic surgery and is not discussed in detail.

The frontalis muscle is considered a muscle of "attention." This thin muscle covers a large portion of the forehead and has no attachments to bone. Its origin is the galea aponeurotica. The muscle insertion is into the procerus, corrugator, orbicularis oculi, and the skin along the superciliary ridge and root of the nose. The action of this muscle is to elevate the eyebrow and wrinkle the forehead. Of clinical note, there is a loose connective tissue surgical plane between the galea and the pericranium that permits ease of dissection during brow-lift surgery.

The frontalis muscle is the main antagonist of the eyebrow depressors. It is supplied by the temporal branch of the facial nerve. The horizontal forehead creases are the direct result of action of the frontalis. These creases are treated effectively with botulinum toxin type A (Botox; Allergan, Irvine, California) treatment and are minimized as a result of a brow-lift procedure.

The procerus muscle (depressor of the brow)

The procerus muscle, also known as pyramidalis nasi, lies superficial to the nasal bone. Its origin is the fascia over the lower region of the nasal bone and the upper part of the lateral nasal cartilage bilaterally. The muscle insertion is into the skin between the eyebrows and root of the nose. Its primary action is to draw down the medial angle of the eyebrows, which creates transverse wrinkles over the bridge of the nose.

The procerus muscle is one of the most common sites for Botox injections. This treatment can produce a medial brow chemolift and eliminate the glabelar lines associated with aging. The procerus is a small muscle with a large effect on facial cosmesis.

The corrugator supercilii (depressor and adductor of the brow)

The corrugator is a deep muscle located directly against the bone beneath the frontalis and orbicularis oculi muscles. The muscle is just superficial to the supraorbital vessels and nerves. This supraorbital bundle passes deep to the corrugator and turns upward across the orbital rim into the forehead. Its origin is from the medial end of the superciliary arch

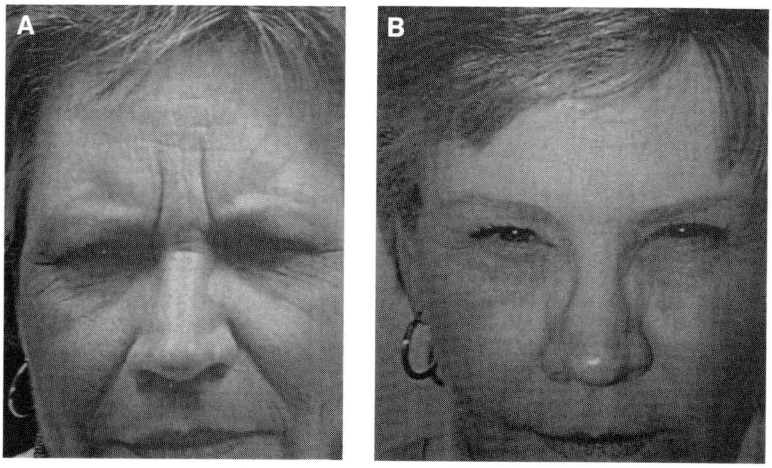

Fig. 3. (*A*) Vertical glabelar wrinkling from activation of corrugator supercilii muscles. (*B*) After successful botulinum toxin injection into the depressors of the brow. (*From* Niamtu J. The use of botulinum toxin in cosmetic facial surgery. Oral Maxillofacial Surg Clin N Am 2000;12(4):601; with permission.)

of the frontal bone close to the nasofrontal suture line. The muscle fibers pass upward and laterally through the fibers of the frontalis and orbicularis oculi to insert into the skin of the medial eyebrow. The action of the corrugator is to draw the eyebrows medially and downward.

Because the corrugator is a depressor and adductor of the brow, it produces vertical glabelar wrinkles (Fig 3A). These lines give a characteristic appearance of anger, frustration, and negative emotion. It is the "frowning" muscle, and may be regarded as the principal muscle in the expression of suffering [1]. This appearance is easily softened with the injection of Botox into this muscle (see Fig. 3B).

The orbicularis oculi (depressor of the brow and the eyelid)

The orbicularis oculi (Fig. 4) is the chief muscle surrounding the orbit. This broad flat muscle occupies the eyelids, covers the supraorbital margins, and overlaps the temporal fossa and cheek region. It functions as the sphincter muscle of the eyelids. The muscle is divided into three major portions: palpebral, orbital, and lacrimal.

The orbital portion is the largest part of the orbicularis oculi. It consists of a series of loops that fan out as they run superiorly and inferiorly about the orbit. These fibers originate and insert on the medial

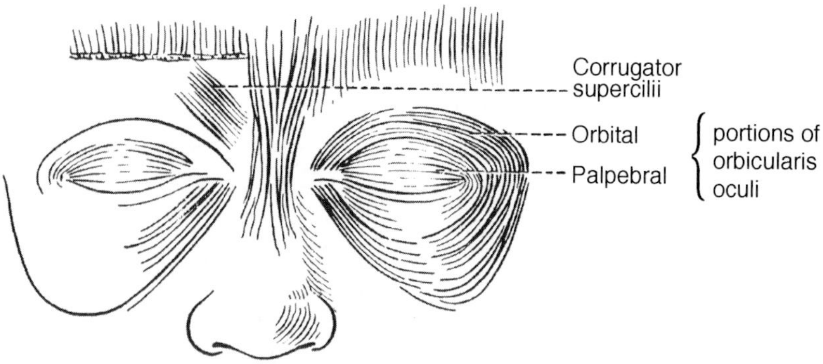

Fig. 4. The orbicularis oculi muscle. (*From* Hollinshead WH. The face. In: Hollinshead WH, editor. Anatomy for surgeons: the head and neck. 3rd edition. Hagerstown, MD: Harper and Row; 1982. p. 297, copyright Philadelphia, PA: Lippincott, William and Wilkins; with permission.)

part of the medial palpebral ligament and the adjacent orbital margin. In addition, the fibers may arise from the nasal portion of the frontal bone and the frontal process of the maxilla. There also can be a lateral insertion into skin. Some of the fibers of the superior medial orbital component function as depressors of the medial brow. The fibers are often termed *depressor supercilii*. The superior lateral orbital orbicularis acts partly as a depressor of the lateral eyebrow [2].

The palpebral portion originates from the bifurcation of the medial palpebral ligament and spreads in concentric curves over the eyelids anterior to the orbital septum [1]. The muscle fibers pass anterior to the tarsal plates and insert laterally into the lateral palpebral raphe (lateral palpebral ligament). The upper and lower portions over the tarsal plates act as a sphincter and, together, act to produce a wink. Acting separately causes blinking. The palpebral portion can also involuntarily aid the flow of tears to keep the cornea moist. The medial palpebral arteries (the larger arteries of the lids) lie deep to this portion at the medial corner of the eye [3].

The lacrimal portion is a small area located behind the medial palpebral ligament and lacrimal sac. It originates from the posterior lacrimal crest and adjacent part of the orbital surface of the lacrimal bone and, passing behind the lacrimal sac, divides into an upper and lower slip that are inserted into the superior and inferior tarsi medial to the puncta lacrimalia [1]. The action of this portion is to tense the tarsal plates and compress the lacrimal sac to assist the flow of tears into the nasolacrimal duct.

Forceful contraction of the orbital component induces concentric folds emanating from the lateral canthus, resulting in lateral canthal lines or "crow's feet." In childhood, crow's feet occur only in dynamic situations (eg, laughter and squinting in bright light). In adulthood, these lines are frequently seen even in facial repose [4]. With time, these periocular lines increase with years of sun exposure and dynamic expression. Botox and laser skin resurfacing are techniques often used to soften and erase these lines.

The levator palpebrae superioris (elevator of the upper eyelid)

As mentioned previously, this muscle is not grouped with the muscles of facial expression but it is responsible for opening the eyelids. This thin and flat muscle originates from the inferior surface of the small wing of the sphenoid where it is separated from the optic foramen by the origin of the superior rectus muscle [1]. The muscle insertion is into the upper eyelid. This muscle is not one of the muscles forming the anulus of Zinn; however, its tendon of origin blends with that of the superior rectus at the periosteal attachments [3]. Unlike the muscles of facial expression, the levator is innervated by the superior division of the oculomotor nerve (third cranial nerve). Paralysis of the levator produces a ptosis of the lid and a disappearance of the superior palpebral fold because the tonus of the muscle is responsible for this fold.

At its origin, the levator palpebrae superioris is narrow and tendinous but becomes broad and fleshy and expands anteriorly into a wide aponeurosis after passing the equator of the eyeball. This aponeurosis splits into three lamellae. The superficial lamella blends with the superior part of the orbital septum and is prolonged over the superior tarsus to the palpebral part of the orbicularis oculi and to the deep surface of the skin of the upper eyelid. The middle lamella, largely made up of nonstriated muscular fibers, is inserted into the superior margin of the superior tarsus. The deepest lamella blends with an expansion from the sheath of the superior rectus and, with it, is attached to the superior fornix of the conjunctiva [1]. The medial and lateral extensions of the aponeurosis are known as horns or cornua. The stronger, lateral one deeply indents the front of the lacrimal gland, dividing it into thin palpebral and thick orbital parts to attach to the marginal (zygomatic, orbital) tubercle between the lateral muscular raphe and the lateral palpebral ligament [3]. The medial horn can be traced with more difficulty to an attachment behind the medial palpebral ligament [3].

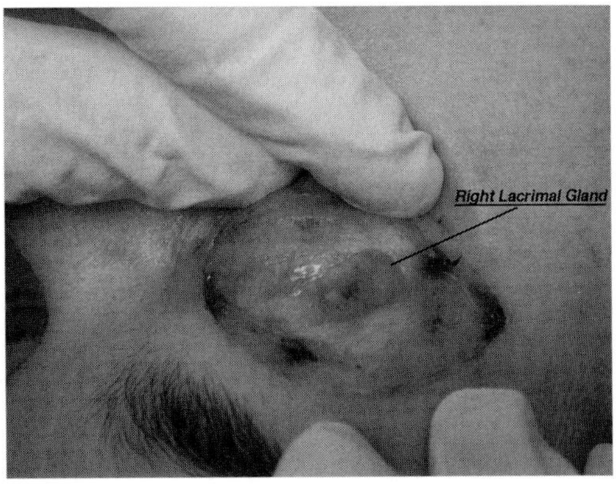

Fig. 5. The lacrimal gland in situ during upper eyelid blepharoplasty of the right eye. (Courtesy of Joseph Niamtu III, DMD, Richmond, Virginia.)

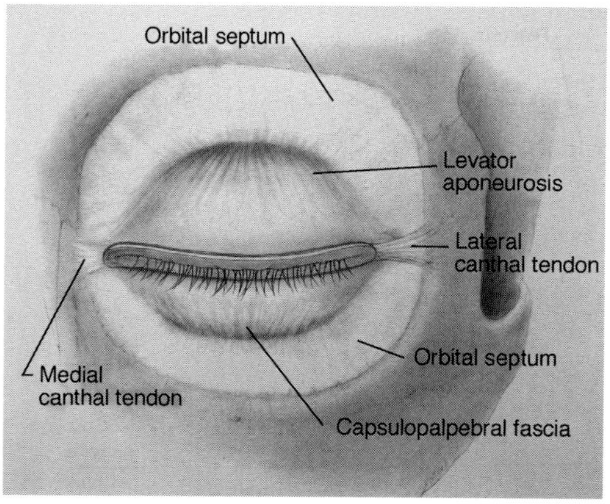

Fig. 6. The levator aponeurosis and the orbital septum. (*From* Putterman AM. Eyelid anatomy. In: Putterman AM, editor. Cosmetic oculoplastic surgery. 2nd edition. Philadelphia, PA: WB Saunders; 1993. p. 76; with permission.)

The superior tarsal (Müller's) muscle is firmly attached to the inferior surface of the levator and passes downward behind the aponeurotic part [3]. This thin sheet of smooth muscle inserts into the upper border of the tarsus. Although the function of this muscle is similar to the levator's function, it should be noted that this muscle is innervated by the sympathetic nervous system.

The levator palpebrae superioris muscle and the lacrimal gland that it divides are key identifiable landmarks during upper-eyelid blepharoplasty (Fig. 5). The levator should be protected when dissecting through the orbital septum during medial and middle fat pad reduction. The levator aponeurosis is identified after dissection through the orbital septum (Fig. 6). The lacrimal gland should not be mistaken for a lateral fat pad and inadvertently removed, which would result in xerophthalmia.

Of clinical note, there are three significant anatomic differences between the Caucasian and Asian populations regarding upper-eyelid blepharoplasty. The Caucasian eyelid is a double eyelid because a superior palpebral fold is created when the lid is opened. The Asian eyelid is a single eyelid because no palpebral fold is formed on eyelid opening. The method of insertion of the levator aponeurosis determines this difference between the two patient populations. Filaments of the levator aponeurosis penetrate the orbital septum and orbicularis oculi in the Caucasian population to insert into the dermis of the upper eyelid (Fig. 7A). In contrast, the levator aponeurosis fibers of the Asian population terminate on the tarsal plate of the upper eyelid without penetrating the orbital septum and orbicularis oculi (see Fig. 7B). Another key difference involves the anatomy of the periorbital fat compartment. In both types of eyelids, the periorbital fat compartment is enclosed by the orbital septum, but in the Asian lid, because of the lack of preseptal adhesions, the periorbital fat compartment descends inferiorly, coursing anterior to the tarsal plate [5]. The more inferior location of periorbital fat and increased amounts of subcutaneous and suborbicularis fat are responsible for the characteristic puffiness of the Asian eyelid [5]. The third difference between Asian and Caucasian upper eyelids is the epicanthal fold, a

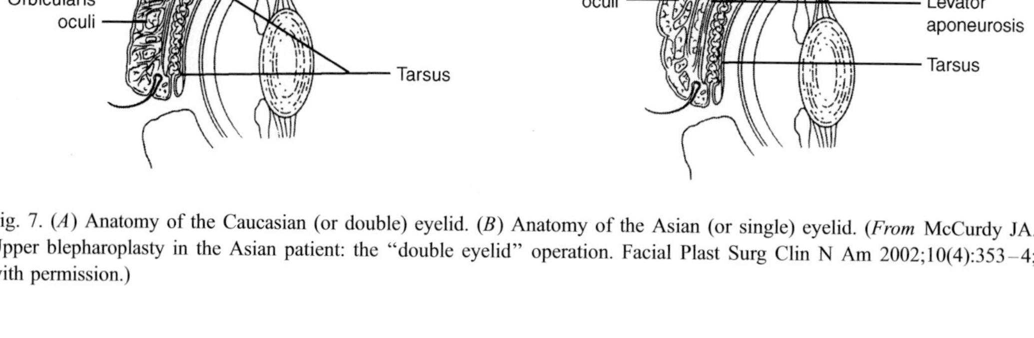

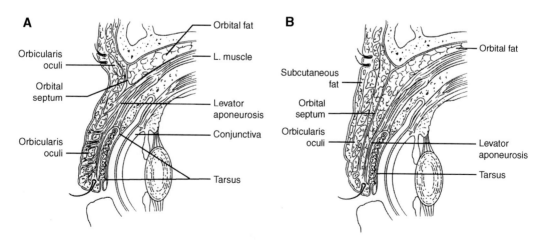

Fig. 7. (*A*) Anatomy of the Caucasian (or double) eyelid. (*B*) Anatomy of the Asian (or single) eyelid. (*From* McCurdy JA. Upper blepharoplasty in the Asian patient: the "double eyelid" operation. Facial Plast Surg Clin N Am 2002;10(4):353–4; with permission.)

structure that is present in approximately 90% of East Asians [5]. Modification of the epicanthus is one of the treatment goals in Asian blepharoplasty.

The musculature of the middle facial third

This group of muscles can be defined by their action on the ears, nose, and mouth. They include the extrinsic muscles of the ear, the muscles of the nose, and the muscles of the mouth. These muscles include the auricularis anterior, auricularis superior, auricularis posterior, nasalis, depressor septi, levator labii superioris alaeque nasi, levator labii superioris, levator anguli oris, zygomaticus major, and zygomaticus minor (Fig. 8A, B). Some of these muscles act as elevators and others act as depressors. Each of these muscles is described in detail along with its relevance to cosmetic facial surgery.

The auricularis muscles (anterior, superior, posterior)

The auricularis anterior (Fig. 9) is the smallest of the three triangular muscles. Its origin is from the anterior part of the deep temporal fascia. The muscle extends downward and slightly backward to insert into the anterior part of the helix. The muscle's action is to draw the ear forward and upward. The muscle is supplied by the temporal branch of the facial nerve.

The auricularis superior (see Fig. 9) is the largest of the three muscles. Lying just behind the anterior,

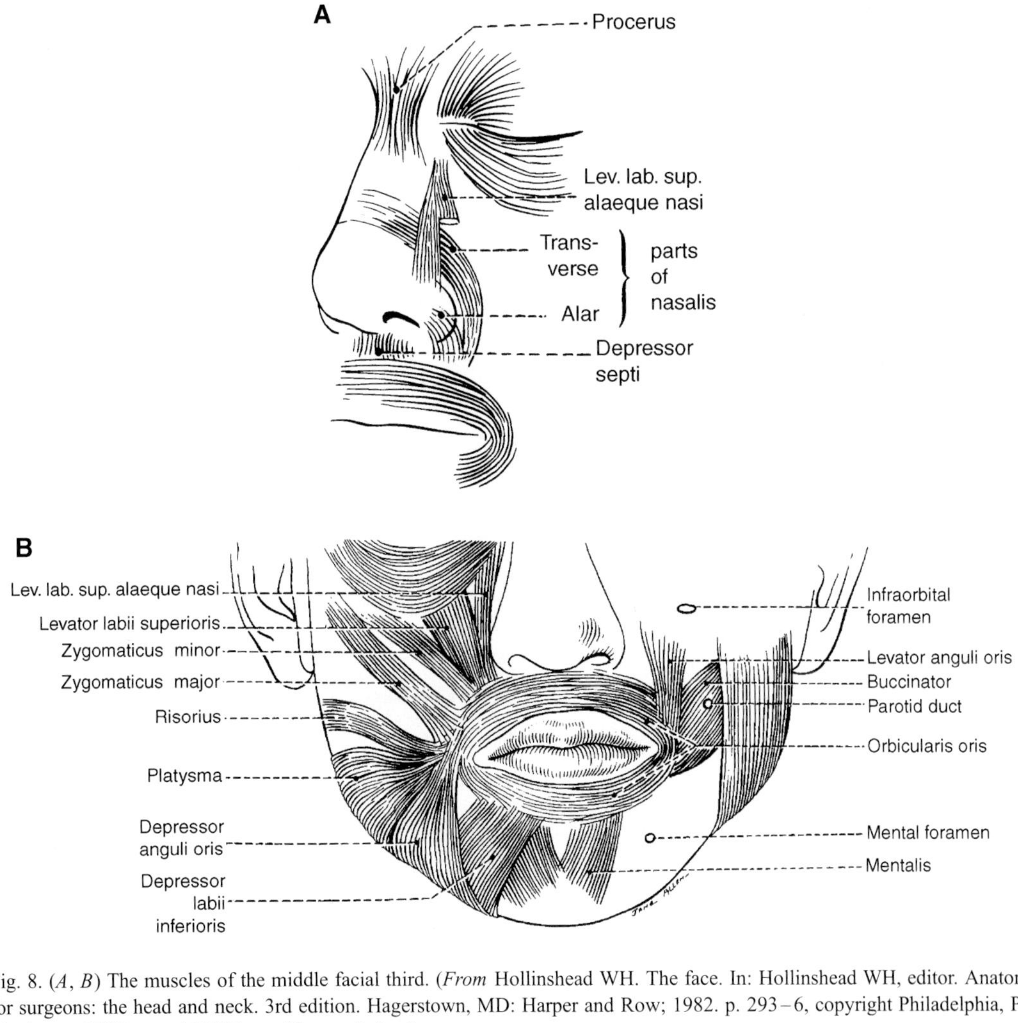

Fig. 8. (*A*, *B*) The muscles of the middle facial third. (*From* Hollinshead WH. The face. In: Hollinshead WH, editor. Anatomy for surgeons: the head and neck. 3rd edition. Hagerstown, MD: Harper and Row; 1982. p. 293–6, copyright Philadelphia, PA: Lippincott, William and Wilkins; with permission.)

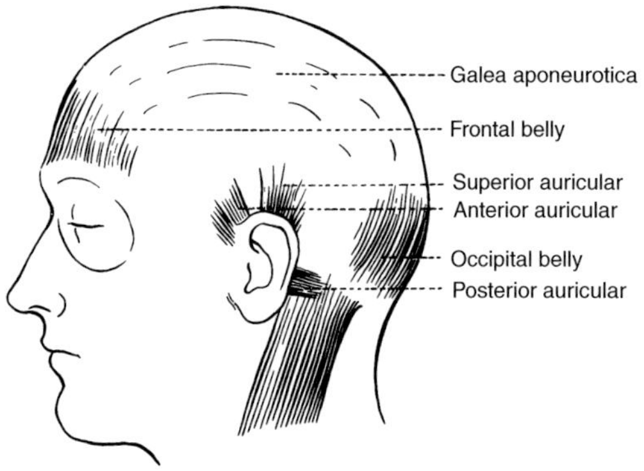

Fig. 9. The auricularis muscles. (*From* Hollinshead WH. The face. In: Hollinshead WH, editor. Anatomy for surgeons: the head and neck. 3rd edition. Hagerstown, MD: Harper and Row; 1982. p. 299, copyright Philadelphia, PA: Lippincott, William and Wilkins; with permission.)

its origin is also from the deep temporal fascia. The muscle descends to insert on the cranial surface of the auricle. The action of this muscle is to elevate the ear. The muscle is supplied by the temporal and posterior auricular branches of the facial nerve.

The auricularis posterior (see Fig. 9) originates from the base of the mastoid process of the temporal bone. The muscle extends over the insertion of the sternocleidomastoid muscle to insert on the convexity of the cranial surface of the concha. The action of this muscle allows us to draw our ears backward. The muscle is supplied by the posterior auricular branch of the facial nerve.

These three muscles vary considerably in development. The anterior and superior auricular muscles act as ear elevators. Some individuals can use them to execute voluntary movements of the auricle [1]. Their relevance to cosmetic facial surgery is limited, except when discussing otoplasty.

The nasalis muscle (dilator and compressor of the nares)

The nasalis (Fig. 10) is the best-developed muscle in the nasal group. This muscle consists of two parts: transverse and alar. The transverse part (compressor naris) originates from the canine eminence of the maxilla. Its fibers proceed upward and medially, expanding into a thin aponeurosis and inserting with that of the muscle of the opposite side and with the aponeurosis of the procerus across the bridge of the nose. The transverse part of the nasalis depresses the cartilaginous part of the nose and draws the ala toward the septum.

The alar part (dilator naris) originates from the subnasal fossa of the maxilla above the lateral incisor tooth medial to the transverse part. The muscle inserts into the lower part of the cartilaginous ala of the nose. The alar part of the nasalis enlarges the aperture of the nares. Its action in ordinary breathing is to resist

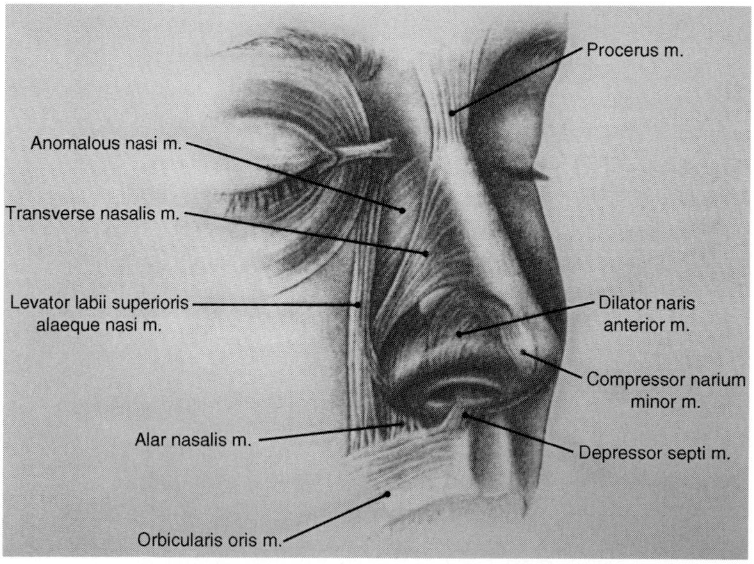

Fig. 10. The nasal muscles of facial expression. (*From* Oneal RM, Beil RJ, Schlesinger J. Surgical anatomy of the nose. Otolaryngolog Clin N Am 1999;32(1):149; with permission.)

the tendency of the nostrils to close from atmospheric pressure. In difficult breathing and in some emotions (ie, anger), it contracts strongly [1].

The upper portion of the nasalis muscle contracts and produces radial lines at the radix of the nose [4]. These upper nasalis lines, or "bunny lines," can be softened successfully with the application of 3 to 5 units (U) of Botox on each side [4]. Care should be taken to not inject too low in the nasofacial groove, which can weaken the levator labii superioris alaeque nasi and levator labii superioris, producing aesthetically significant ipsilateral lip ptosis and creating an unpleasant aesthetic effect [4].

The depressor septi (depressor of the nose)

The depressor septi (see Fig. 10) originates from the subnasal fossa of the maxilla. Its fibers extend upward to be inserted into the septum and the posterior part of the ala of the nose [3]. At its origin, it lies deep to the orbicularis oris [3]. The muscle acts to draw the ala of the nose downward, thereby constricting the aperture of the nares [1]. This muscle is innervated by the buccal branch of the facial nerve. Its relevance to cosmetic facial surgery is limited.

The levator labii superioris alaeque nasi (elevator of lip; dilator of nares)

This narrow muscle originates from the frontal process of the maxilla alongside the nose (see Fig. 10). The muscle divides into two slips. One slip inserts into the skin and greater alar cartilage of the nose. The other major portion passes obliquely downward, blending with the levator labii superioris, to insert into the skin and musculature of the upper lip [3]. This muscle's action is responsible for raising the upper lip and dilating the nare.

As mentioned previously, it is important to avoid injecting Botox into this muscle for the wrong reasons, as it could result in temporary lip ptosis and an unpleasant outcome. Very small amounts of Botox, however, have been injected into the levator labii superioris alaeque nasi muscle to drop the upper lip in the treatment of maxillary gingival excess on smiling.

The levator labii superioris (elevator of the lip)

The levator labii superioris is a thin quadrangular muscle that takes a broad origin from the lower margin of the orbit immediately above the infraorbital foramen of the maxilla under cover of the orbicularis oculi. Some of its fibers are attached to the maxilla; others are attached to the zygomatic bone [1]. Its fibers converge to mingle with the orbicularis oris and insert into the skin of the lateral half of the upper lip between the levator anguli oris and the levator labii superioris alaeque nasi. The muscle acts by everting and elevating the upper lip.

Vertical lines in the midface (also known as melolabial folds) give an impression of hostility, fatigue, and age [4]. Weakening the levator labii superioris with 1 to 2 U of Botox can soften the upper half of the fold but at the price of causing ptosis of the upper lip [4]. Most middle-aged patients are already concerned about the elongation of their cutaneous upper lip (and narrowing of the vermilion); therefore, this treatment has not been popular [4].

The levator anguli oris (elevator of angle of the mouth)

The levator anguli oris lies more deeply than the other levator muscles and the zygomaticus muscles. The muscle originates from the canine fossa of the maxilla, immediately below the infraorbital foramen. The muscle fibers run downward to the corner of the mouth and insert into the angle of the mouth. The muscle intermingles with both the zygomaticus major and the depressor anguli oris, and sends fasciculi around the corner of the mouth to blend with the lower part of the orbicularis oris (Fig. 11). The action of this muscle is to deepen the nasolabial furrow during an expression of contempt or disdain. The facial artery runs across the lower part of the muscle. Branches of the infraorbital nerve and vessels spread out in the connective tissue between it and the overlying muscles [3].

The action of the levator anguli oris contributes to the formation of the nasolabial fold. This dynamic wrinkle, which varies in appearance between individuals, has a profound effect on facial aging. Various wrinkle fillers and implants such as Restylane (Q-Med AB, Uppsala, Sweden), Zyderm/Zyplast collagen (McGhan Medical, Santa Barbara, California), Alloderm (Life Cell Corp., The Wood Lands, Texas), Gore-Tex (W.L. Gore, Flagstaff, Arizona), and autologous fat have been used to camouflage a pronounced nasolabial fold.

The zygomaticus major (elevator of the mouth)

The zygomaticus major is a superficially located, ribbonlike muscle, which passes superficial to the masseter and buccinator muscles and to the facial vein and artery [3]. This muscle originates from the zygomatic bone, in front of the zygomaticotemporal

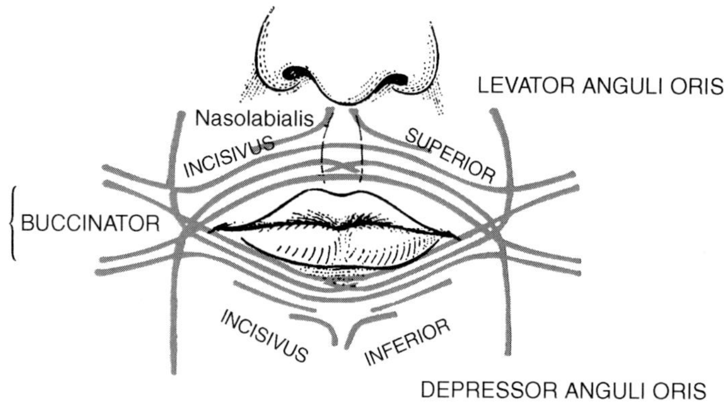

Fig. 11. Diagram showing arrangement of fibers of orbicularis oris muscle. (*From* Clemente CD. Muscles and fasciae. In: Clemente CD, editor. Gray's anatomy. 30th American edition. Philadelphia: Lea and Febiger; 1985. p. 445, copyright Philadelphia, PA: Lippincott, William and Wilkins; with permission.)

suture. It passes obliquely downward and forward to insert into the skin and mucosa of the corner of the mouth. The muscle's action is to draw the mouth upward and laterally, as in laughing.

The zygomaticus major works in conjunction with the levator anguli oris to raise the angle of the mouth and form the nasolabial fold. The treatment of this area was previously mentioned.

The zygomaticus minor (elevator of the mouth)

The zygomaticus minor originates from the malar surface of the zygomatic bone, anterior to the origin of the zygomaticus major. It runs toward the mouth almost parallel to the zygomaticus major to insert into the skin and mucosa of the upper lip just medial to the corner of the mouth. The muscle acts to elevate and evert the upper lip.

Incidentally, the zygomaticus minor is not present in 25% of individuals [4]. Unlike the zygomaticus major, it is not considered part of the modiolus at the angle of the mouth. The zygomaticus major and minor muscles are direct antagonists of the depressor anguli oris muscle, which has cosmetic implications that are covered when reviewing the depressor anguli oris.

The musculature of the lower facial third

This group of muscles can be defined primarily by their action on the lips and lower face. They include the lower group of mouth muscles and the platysma muscle in the neck, which belongs to the facial group. These muscles are the risorius, orbicularis oris, buccinator, depressor labii inferioris, depressor anguli oris, mentalis, and platysma (see Fig. 12). Some of these muscles act as elevators and others act as depressors. Each of these muscles is described in detail along with its relevance to cosmetic facial surgery.

The risorius (lateral retractor of angle of mouth)

The risorius muscle is unique. It differs from most of the facial muscles in that it does not arise from bone. The muscle originates from the subcutaneous tissue over the parotid gland (also known as parotid-masseteric fascia). It is a thin, usually poorly developed muscle, lying at about the upper border of the facial portion of the platysma, partly overlapping this superficially and often separable from it without difficulty [3]. The risorius runs forward and slightly downward, across the masseter muscle to insert into the skin and mucosa of the corner of the mouth. This muscle crosses superficial to the facial vein and artery [3]. The muscle action of the risorius is to retract the angle of the mouth, as in grinning. The risorius is innervated by the buccal branch of the facial nerve.

This muscle, when grouped with the other muscles of the modiolus, also contributes to the formation of the nasolabial fold. The modiolus and its effect on the aging process are reviewed in the following sections.

The buccinator (principal muscle of the cheek)

Buccinator comes from a Latin term for trumpet player [5]. As in blowing a trumpet, when the cheeks are distended with air, the buccinators compress them and force the air out between the lips [1]. The

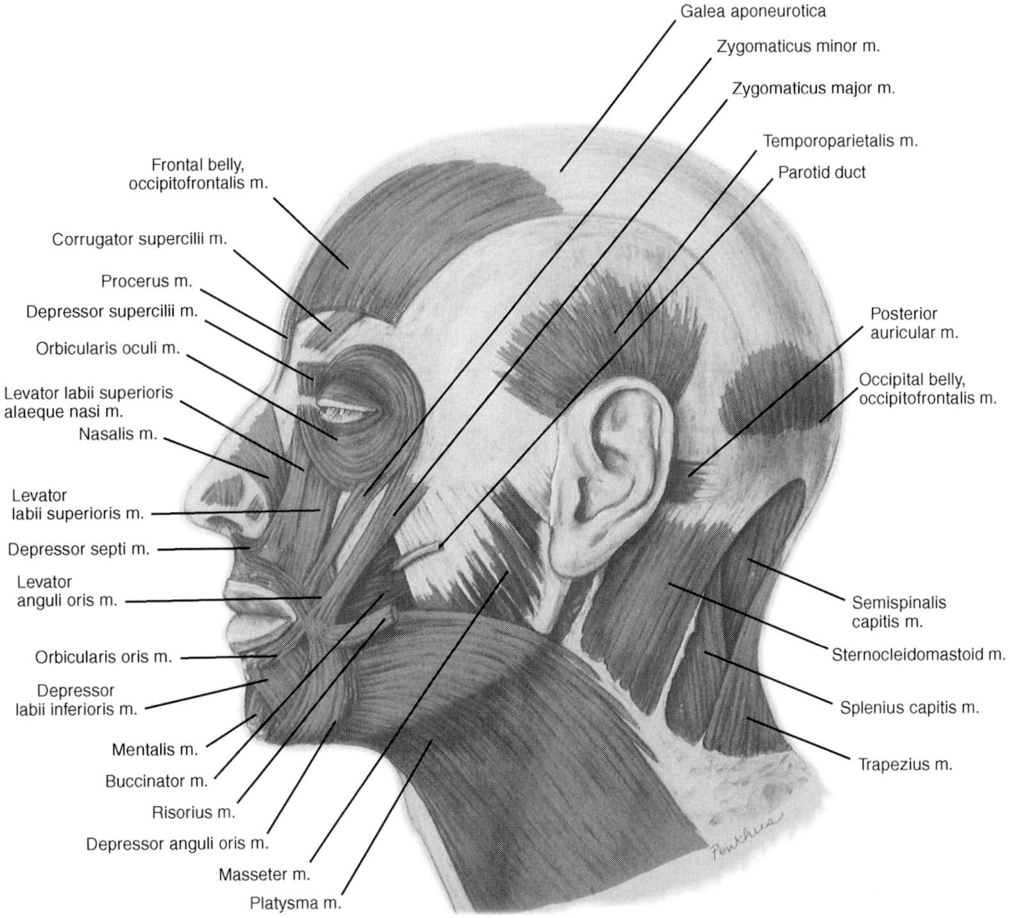

Fig. 12. Superficial muscles of the face, scalp, and neck. Left lateral view. (*From* Clemente CD. Muscles and fasciae. In: Clemente CD, editor. Gray's anatomy. 30th American edition. Philadelphia: Lea and Febiger; 1985. p. 440, copyright Lippincott, William and Wilkins; with permission.)

buccinator, quadrangular in form, lies deeper than the other facial muscles. Located lateral to the teeth, it forms the lateral wall of the oral cavity.

Anatomically, the buccinator is unique. It has three origins. One origin from above is the alveolar process of the maxilla, opposite the molar teeth. Another origin from below is the alveolar process of the mandible, opposite the molar teeth. From behind, the muscle originates from the pterygomandibular raphe, which sits between the buccinator and the superior pharyngeal constrictor muscles. The function of the lips is supported by the pattern of insertion of the buccinator. The upper fibers pass into the upper lip to become continuous with the orbicularis oris [6]. The middle fibers converge toward the angle of the mouth and decussate, passing to the upper and lower lips to enhance the sphincter action of the orbicularis oris muscle. The lower fibers pass directly into the lower lip to become continuous with the orbicularis oris [6].

The superficial surface of the buccinator is covered by the buccopharyngeal fascia and the buccal fat pad [1]. Its deep surface is adjacent to the buccal glands and the mucous membrane of the mouth [1]. The parotid duct passes forward on the muscle and pierces it to enter the mouth opposite the maxillary second molar tooth. The transverse facial artery roughly parallels the duct, usually lying above it [3]. The buccinator muscle is innervated by the buccal branches of the facial nerve (not through the buccal branch of the mandibular nerve, which also lies on its outer surface and sends twigs through it to the buccal mucosa) [3]. The buccinator is an important accessory muscle of mastication. The muscle acts to hold the food between the teeth during mastication and forces food out of the vestibule before swallowing. As previously mentioned, the muscle also forces air during blowing.

The depressor labii inferioris (depressor of the lip)

This depressor of the lower lip originates from the oblique line of the front of the mandible, between the mental symphysis and the mental foramen. The anterior fibers of the depressor anguli oris partially cover the muscle. The depressor labii inferioris passes upward in front of the mental foramen (the fiber bundles running medially) and is inserted into the skin and mucous membrane of the lower lip [3]. Its fibers blend with the orbicularis oris and the depressor labii inferioris of the opposite side. At its origin, it is continuous with the fibers of the platysma, and considerable fat is intermingled with the fibers of this muscle [1]. This muscle's action draws the lower lip directly downward and somewhat laterally, producing the expression of irony [1].

The depressor anguli oris (depressor of the angle of the mouth)

This triangularis muscle is usually well developed. It originates from the external oblique line of the mandible lateral to and below the depressor labii inferioris. At its origin, the posterior border of this muscle is continuous with upper fibers of the platysma [3]. The depressor anguli oris muscle fibers converge to the corner of the mouth. They are partly inserted into the skin and mucous membrane of the lips and partly become continuous with the orbicularis oris, the risorius, and the fibers of the levator anguli oris. The muscle acts to depress the angle of the mouth, being the antagonist of the levator anguli oris and zygomaticus major [1]. Acting with the levator anguli oris, it draws the angle of the mouth medially [1]. This muscle is innervated by the marginal mandibular and lower buccal branches of the facial nerve.

Some people have persistent vertical grooves at the lateral corners of the mouth (also known as mandibulolabial folds or "drool lines"), giving an impression of fixed disapproval or sadness. Persistent contraction of the depressor anguli oris bends the corners of the mouth into an expression of fixed disapproval [4]. By selective chemodenervation of the depressor anguli oris with Botox, the zygomaticus muscles become relatively unopposed as elevators of the corners of the mouth, so that the mouth corners assume a more relaxed neutral position [4]. Carruthers and Carruthers [4] have recommended 2 to 5 U of Botox per muscle, depending on the size of the individual muscle.

The orbicularis oris (sphincter muscle of the mouth)

The orbicularis oris is a complex sphincter muscle. To what extent true sphincteric fibers actually exist is not known [3]. Its primary origin is from many neighboring muscles and the subnasal and incisive fossae. The muscle inserts into the skin and mucous membrane of the lips.

There are 10 pairs of surrounding muscles whose fibers become continuous with the orbicularis oris [6]. Some fibers of the orbicularis oris are derived from other facial muscles that insert into the lips, whereas other fibers are intrinsic to the muscle itself [6]. The orbicularis oris consists of four strata of muscular fibers surrounding the orifice of the mouth and coursing in different directions [1]. The deepest stratum includes the incisivus labii superioris and inferioris, which are attached to the maxilla and mandible, respectively. The buccinator muscle forms the next stratum. Some of the buccinator fibers—namely, those near the middle of the muscle—decussate at the angle of the mouth. Those arising from the maxilla pass to the lower lip, and those from the mandible pass to the upper lip [1]. The uppermost and lowermost fibers, derived from the buccinator, pass across the lips from side to side without decussation [1]. Superficial to the buccinator is another layer, formed on each side by fibers from the levator and depressor anguli oris muscles that cross each other at the angle of the mouth [1]. These muscles pass into opposite lips and are inserted into the skin at the midline: those from the levator anguli oris pass to the lower lip, and those from the depressor anguli oris pass to the upper lip [1]. The most superficial stratum comes from the other muscles surrounding the mouth.

The orbicularis oris contains the insertions of many of the muscles already described as reaching the upper and lower lips [3]. Through the action of the whole and the various parts, the orbicularis oris draws the lips together, draws inward the corners of the lips, and either purses them or draws them against the teeth [3]. The orbicularis oris is innervated by the buccal branches of the facial nerve.

The dynamic action of the orbicularis oris in combination with photoaged skin or smoking can lead to the formation of vertical lip rhytides. These unsightly wrinkles are especially troublesome after the application of lipstick. The lipstick tends to run into these lines, resulting in vertical color bands surrounding the oral cavity. Local microinjection of Botox causes segmental weakening of the lip sphincter, relaxing the folds and allowing the lip to appear "pseudoeverted" and smoother [4]. Carruthers and Carruthers [4] usually inject 1 U per fold, to a maximum of 1 to 2 U per hemilip. This procedure is an effective adjunctive treatment to perioral carbon dioxide laser skin resurfacing. Care should be taken to inform the patient that this treatment causes mild compromise to the sphincter action of the orbicularis oris.

The mentalis (elevator of lower lip and skin of chin)

The mentalis is the deeper-lying muscle of the lower oral group of muscles. It originates from the incisive fossa of the mandible at the level of the root of the lower lateral incisor. The two muscle bellies diverge from the incisive fossa, passing downward to their insertion into the integument of the chin. A small column of adipose tissue usually separates these two muscles in the midline. This short, stout muscle is placed deep to the depressor labii inferioris [3]. In contrast to the other mouth muscles, the mentalis is the only one that does not insert into the orbicularis oris muscle. Also unique to this muscle is the fact that its action is opposite in direction to the other muscles of facial expression [5]. The mentalis acts to raise and protrude the lower lip while wrinkling and elevating the skin of the chin, as in pouting or expressing doubt or disdain [1]. The muscle is innervated by the marginal mandibular branch of the facial nerve.

Botox can be used to treat a deep labiomental fold or the "peau d'orange" chin dimpling (Fig. 13A, B) seen in patients with an overactive mentalis muscle. Carruthers and Carruthers [4] inject 5 to 10 U of Botox into the mentalis at its most distal point (the mentum) from the orbicularis oris, and then massage this area to help it diffuse in the muscle.

The platysma (depressor of the lip)

The platysma is located in the neck, but its primary function is on the face and mandible. This broad sheet of muscle lies in the substance of the superficial fascia of the neck covering the superior parts of the pectoralis major and deltoid muscles. The muscle takes its origin from this fascia covering these muscles. Similar to the risorius muscle, the platysma does not arise from bone. Its fibers ascend over the clavicle, and proceed obliquely upward and medially along the side of the neck [1]. The most anterior fibers interlace across the midline with those of the muscle of the opposite side [1]. The posterior fibers cross the border of the mandible superficial to the facial vessels, and some are inserted into the lower border of the body of the mandible. Other fibers insert into the skin and subcutaneous tissue of the angle of the mouth [6]. Some of these latter fibers blend with some of the muscles connected with the lower lip, especially the depressor anguli oris (triangularis) [3]. Under cover of the platysma, the external jugular vein descends from the angle of the mandible to the clavicle [1]. The platysma's action is to draw the lower lip and corner of the mouth laterally and inferiorly, partially opening the mouth, as in an expression of surprise or horror [1]. When all the fibers act maximally, the skin over the clavicle is wrinkled and drawn toward the mandible, increasing the diameter of the neck, as is seen during the intensive respiration of a sprinting runner [1]. The platysma is innervated by the cervical branch of the facial nerve, the lowest and the least important branch of the facial nerve [3].

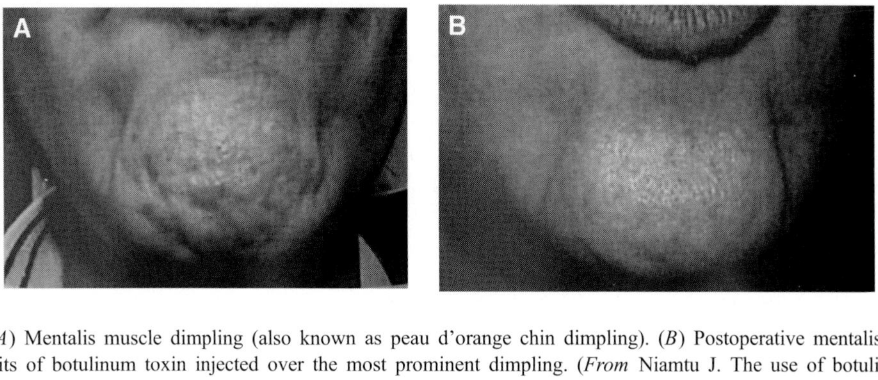

Fig. 13. (*A*) Mentalis muscle dimpling (also known as peau d'orange chin dimpling). (*B*) Postoperative mentalis treatment with 2 units of botulinum toxin injected over the most prominent dimpling. (*From* Niamtu J. The use of botulinum toxin in cosmetic facial surgery. Oral Maxillofacial Surg Clin N Am 2000;12(4):608; with permission.)

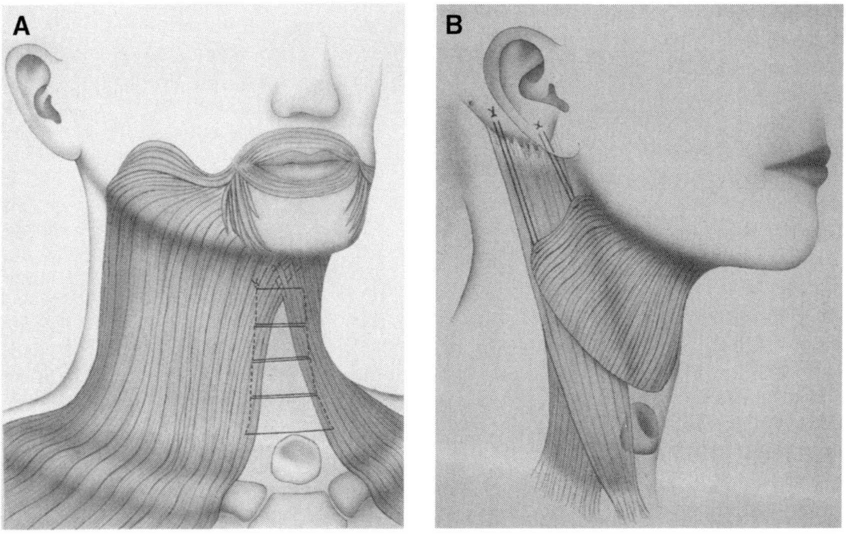

Fig. 14. (*A*) Example of an anterior platysmaplasty. (*B*) Posterior platysma plication with suspension sutures to mastoid periosteum. (*From* Toft KM, Blackwell KE, Keller GS. Submentoplasty: an anatomical approach. Facial Plast Surg Clin N Am 2000;8(2):188–9; with permission.)

The anatomic form of the platysma shows great variability between individuals. The muscle may be composed of delicate, pale, scattered fasciculi, or may form a broad layer of dark robust fibers [1]. It may be deficient or reach well below the clavicle, and it may extend into the face for a short distance or may continue as high as the zygoma [1]. These gross differences in platysmal anatomy from person to person can affect the surgical outcome when trying to rejuvenate the aging neck, depending on which procedure is chosen. During neck dissection, cosmetic surgeons may find a thick robust platysma or a thin and fragile one.

The role of the platysma muscle in cosmetic surgery of the head and neck cannot be overstated. In fact, concern over the aging neck is one of the most common reasons for consultation with a cosmetic surgeon [7]. Correction of neck laxity has been considered to be an integral part of what is currently considered traditional face-lift surgery [7]. Various techniques have been developed to treat the aging neck with or without a face-lift, and most of these involve direct dissection of the platysma muscle. Some form of anterior platysmaplasty is frequently performed in conjunction with liposuction of the neck (Fig. 14A). In fact, the surgical decisions regarding the treatment of this area is one of the most variable among cosmetic surgeons. There is no unanimity of opinion regarding the management of the anterior platysma [7]. Unless the surgeon elects to perform a skin-only face-lift, posterior platysma plication is also a common procedure during face-lift surgery (see Fig. 14B).

Patient variability on presentation includes age, neck laxity, skin quality, presence or absence of anterior platysmal bands, degree of fat accumulation, presence or absence of microgenia, and presence or absence of ptosis of the submandibular gland. Every cosmetic surgeon identifies with the appropriate surgical management of the platysma, not only for its importance during surgical dissection and its relationship to adjacent structures but also for its relevance in determining a successful surgical outcome.

The musculature of the modiolus

The modiolus (Fig. 15) has an influence on youth and beauty in its relationship to the nasolabial fold. It shapes the inferior level of the face, and thus individualizes it from the middle face [8]. German anatomists in the nineteenth century described the modiolus as a definitive muscular formation they named *Knoten* [8]. In the 1920s, Lightoller took this German concept and renamed it "modiolus," insisting on the physiologic interest of this anatomic structure and comparing the modiolus to the "nave of a wheel" and the muscles ending in it to the "radiating spokes of an imaginary wheel" [8]. The modiolus is located lateral to the corner of the mouth at approximately the crown of the maxillary second

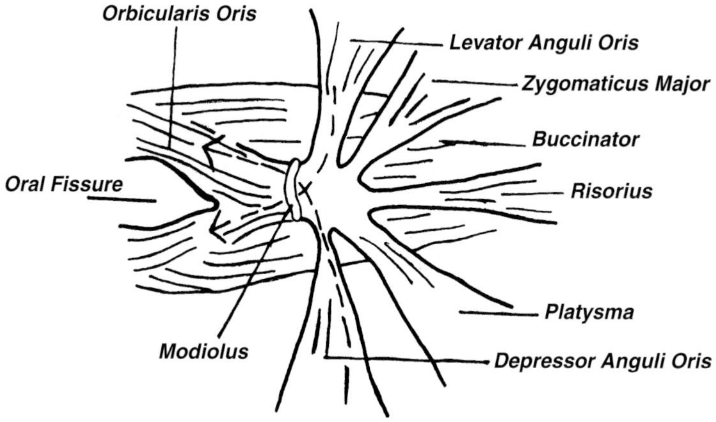

Fig. 15. The muscles of the modiolus.

premolar tooth [6]. It is an area where five muscles are inserted and bound by connective tissue to the buccinator muscle [6]. The exact definition of the modiolus and its macroscopic nature is the "decussation of muscle fibers converging toward and diverging from it" [8]. The five muscles of the modiolus are the levator anguli oris, zygomaticus major, risorius, depressor anguli oris, and platysma.

The cheekbone and modiolus are intimately associated and act together like a dynamic of soft tissues. Their articulation represents the nasolabial fold [8]. Zufferey [8] described the relationship of the nasolabial fold to the modiolus. He stated that some observations are constant even though nasolabial folds can be different from person to person. His observations included "a long convex nasolabial fold is always present with a weak trophic modiolus, and a short concave nasolabial fold is always present with a large trophic modiolus" [8]. Therefore, according to Zufferey [8], the difference between a long convex fold and a short concave fold resides in the muscular trophicity of a patient's modiolus. Clearly, this highlights the interaction of the modiolus and nasolabial fold and their relationship to the degree of facial aging. Most patients seeking consultation with a cosmetic surgeon have the convex form, usually with excess skin above the fold.

Summary

Surgeons are performing more cosmetic surgery today than ever before. The public awareness is high and baby boomers are fueling a cosmetic renaissance. It is important for us to deliver these "goods" safely and effectively. A thorough knowledge of facial anatomy is essential to providing consistent and satisfying results for the patient and the surgeon. Many injectables have become available over the last decade, and thousands of surgical procedures are being performed on a daily basis. These procedures manipulate the facial musculature in one way, shape, or form. With a concise understanding of the muscles of facial expression, the surgeon can perform these procedures with the confidence and skill necessary to achieve successful results for his or her patients.

References

[1] Clemente CD. Muscles and fasciae. In: Clemente CD, editor. Gray's anatomy. 30th American edition. Philadelphia: Lea and Febiger; 1985. p. 438–47.

[2] Zimbler MS, Kokoska MS, Thomas JR. Anatomy and pathophysiology of facial aging. Facial Plast Surg Clin N Am 2001;9(2):179–87.

[3] Hollinshead WH. The face. In: Hollinshead WH, editor. In: Anatomy for surgeons: the head and neck. 3rd edition. Hagerstown, MD: Harper and Row; 1982. p. 292–9.

[4] Carruthers J, Carruthers A. Botulinum toxin (Botox) chemodenervation for facial rejuvenation. Facial Plast Surg Clin N Am 2001;9(2):197–204.

[5] McCurdy JA. Upper blepharoplasty in the Asian patient: the "double eyelid" operation. Facial Plast Surg Clin N Am 2002;10(4):351–68.

[6] Saracco CG, Crabill EV. The muscles of facial expression. The head and neck. Pittsburgh, PA: University of Pittsburgh School of Dental Medicine Syllabus; 1994. p. 117–27.

[7] Tobin HA. Treatment of the aging neck. Oral Maxillofacial Surg Clin N Am 2000;12(4):709–17.

[8] Zufferey JA. Importance of the modiolus in plastic surgery. Plast Reconstr Surg 2002;110(1):331–4.

ELSEVIER
SAUNDERS

Oral Maxillofacial Surg Clin N Am 17 (2005) 17 – 28

ORAL AND MAXILLOFACIAL SURGERY CLINICS of North America

New Lip and Wrinkle Fillers

Joseph Niamtu III, DMD

Oral/Maxillofacial and Cosmetic Facial Surgery, 10230 Cherokee Road, Richmond, VA 23235, USA

One of the most requested cosmetic procedures is enhancement of the lips. Since the beginning of time, humans have adorned their lips in many ways for reasons including courtship, social status, and beauty (Fig. 1).

It has been said that the lips are the only exposed sexual organ in our society. There is no doubt that lips play an important part in sexual attraction and lovemaking. In today's female Hollywood elite, it seems that one's prowess is directly proportional to lip size. Some actresses such as Julia Roberts, Angelina Jolie, and Goldie Hawn are even defined by their lips. Lip accentuation comes and goes with changing fashions. A 1950s picture of Elizabeth Taylor or Marilyn Monroe is sure to show large, red lips, whereas a 1960s picture of Twiggy or Barbara Streisand may show thin, barely colored lips. What is constant is the fact that attractive lips are a mainstay in the esthetic appreciation of female and male beauty.

What makes an esthetic lip is defined differently for different races and cultures. Volume, pout, outline, and vermilion exposure are key elements of beauty. As is true for other anatomy, some people are simply born with beautiful lips. They have larger lips with a wide smile, their lips project more in profile, they have sharply angulated contours, and they show a larger amount of vermilion than the average person (Fig. 2A–C).

In general, the esthetic upper lip is one third of the total lip mass and the lower lip represents a larger structure, with two thirds of the total lip height. The outline of the upper lip is termed *Cupid's bow* and is defined by the angulated mucocutaneous junction. Some individuals exhibit a rounded Cupid's bow, whereas others have very angulated lines. The outline of the vermilion/cutaneous junction in the upper lip is the shape of an "M" and is curvilinear in the lower lip (Fig. 3).

The "white roll" is described as a linear protrubence that follows Cupid's bow in the upper lip. This subtle but important area produces the light reflex above the vermilion/cutaneous junction, calling attention to the fine outline. In addition, this area outlines the lips and, in the lateral view, adds to the pout of the attractive lip.

Aging causes thinning of the lips. The senescent lip is also reduced in volume by the loss of vertical dimension from occlusial attrition.

The key to enhancing the lips is to give the patient what nature did not or to accentuate the existing anatomy. In the author's practice, only one man has sought lip enhancement with fillers over a 20-year period. Basically, 100% of lip filler injection is performed in Caucasian women between the ages of 30 and 75 years. Although the most common request for fillers is in the lips, fillers can be used in a multitude of other cosmetic facial applications and are discussed in this article.

Facial fillers

Over the millennia, various substances have been injected into the face, including wax, silicone, and animal products [1,2]. Contemporary cosmetic facial surgery includes many options to augment lips, folds, and wrinkles. For decades, bovine collagen has been the "gold standard" for facial filler augmentation in the United States [3]. Our European, Canadian, and Australian neighbors have been more proactive in the use of various fillers [4]; this technology is just reaching our shores and, in part,

E-mail address: niamtu@niamtu.com

1042-3699/05/$ – see front matter
doi:10.1016/j.coms.2004.10.001

oralmaxsurgery.theclinics.com

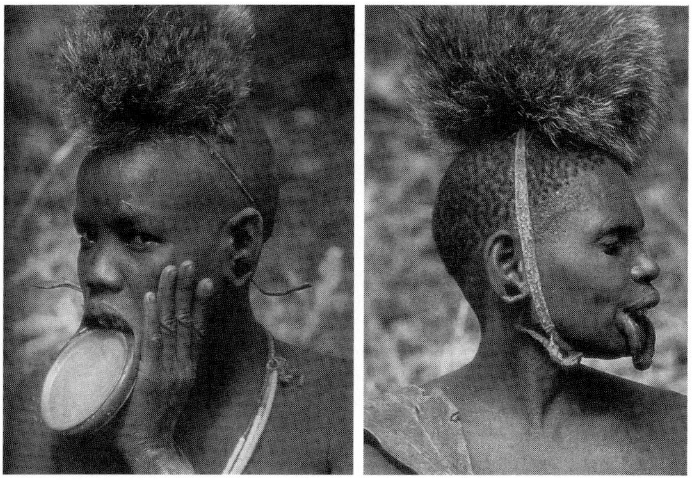

Fig. 1. An African native shows the extent that some societies have gone to call attention to the lips.

is responsible for the enormous media coverage of injectable filler substances.

An overview of injectable filler substances can be confusing. There exist many options, many fillers, many substances, many materials, and many claims of superiority. As stated earlier, bovine collagen (Zyplast, Zyderm; Inamed Corp., Santa Barbara, California) dominated the United States market for over 2 decades. Because these products were of bovine derivation, allergy testing was a prerequisite. Classically, patients were inoculated in the forearm with the material and, if no local allergic response was seen at 30 days, then the material was assumed safe. The need for testing proved to be a great

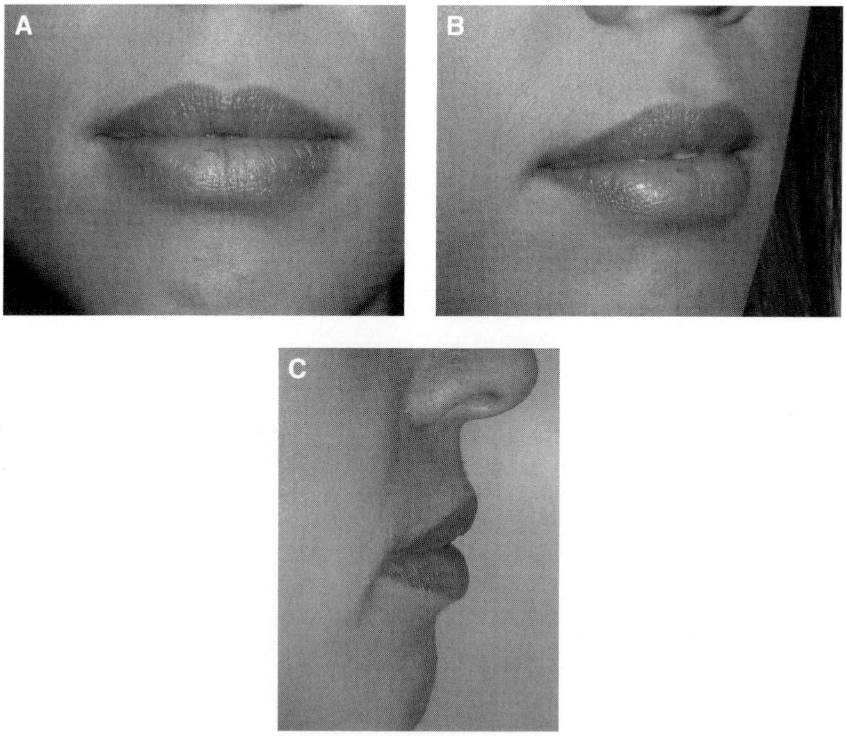

Fig. 2. (*A–C*) Esthetic lips are a function of volume, projection, contour angulation, and vermilion exposure.

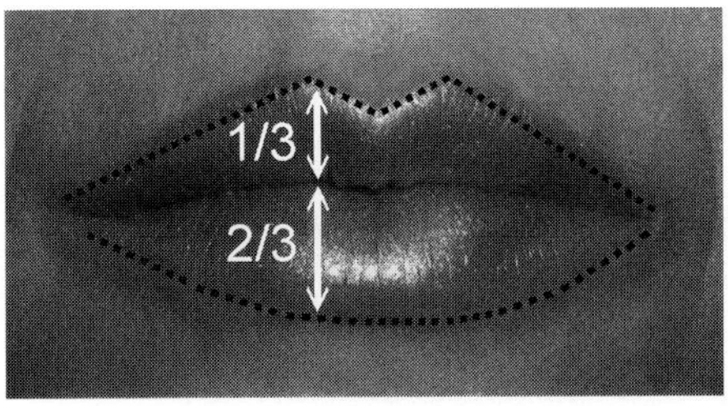

Fig. 3. The M configuration of Cupid's bow and the relative size of the upper and lower lips are shown.

drawback because many cosmetic consumers are spontaneous and want immediate treatment. There has been a foreign invasion of injectable fillers since December 2003. Hyaluronic acid (Restylane; Medicis, Scottsdale, Arizona), which has been used in many countries for over a decade, received Food and Drug Administration (FDA) approval in the United States (Fig. 4). This marketing release brought an onslaught of media attention that boosted the entire perception of and desire for fillers by the aging baby boomers.

Restylane changed the paradigm for injectable fillers for numerous reasons. First, it is a nonanimal product (hyaluronic acid is a naturally occurring substance in humans [4]), which means that there is no reason for allergy testing, one of the biggest drawbacks of bovine collagen products. Second, studies showed that Restylane lasts longer than Zyplast. The longevity of Zyplast has long been a problem for patients. Although the product was easy to use and produced an excellent result, it lasted only several months in most patients, whereas some studies showed Restylane can last up to 8 months [5,6]. One of the reasons for the extended longevity with Restylane is a process called isovolemic degradation. Normally, collagen fillers are simply phagocytized and degraded, which causes decrease in volume. Hyaluronic acid undergoes isovolemic degradation. In this process, water is drawn into the filler molecule as the filler degrades. By doing this, the filler volume is retained longer as more water is continually drawn into the filler molecule (Fig. 5) [7]. Multiple studies have shown Restylane to be a safe and effective facial filler [8,9].

In 2003, Inamed introduced Cosmoplast and Cosmoderm, which are human collagen derivatives produced from human foreskin. Because these products are of nonanimal origin, allergy testing is not necessary. Although these products are very easy to inject because they have excellent flow properties, the author has found them to posses the same longevity as the bovine collagen predecessors. Hyaluron (Inamed) gained FDA approval in 2004 and competes with Restylane in the new filler arena. Although the author has little experience with Hyaluron, differences lie in the fact that this hyaluronic acid product is derived from animals (rooster combs) and contains less hyaluronic acid per milliliter than Restylane.

Oral and maxillofacial surgeons have used hydroxyapetite products for augmentation for the past 20 years. Radiance FN (BioForm, Franksville, Wisconsin) is an injectable filler that consists of hydroxyapatite microspheres in a soluble gel vehicle (Fig. 6) [10].

The use of Radiance FN in cosmetic facial augmentation is off-label because the FDA approval for his product is for vocal cord plumping and as a radiopaque soft tissue marker. The author uses Radiance FN when requested by patients, primarily in the nasolabial folds and lips. The flow properties of Radiance FN are different from other fillers. The most noticeable property of Radiance FN is that a little product goes a long way. Because this product is hydroxyapetite based, the longevity is measured in years, not months. For this reason, overfill or asymmetry can be a huge problem because it persists for a long time. The author does not recommend this product for the novice injector. Extreme care must be used to not cause lumpiness, overfill, or asymmetry. In general, the author uses 0.2 mL on each lip quadrant at a single sitting so as to not overfill. The patients are then seen several weeks later to see whether touch-up is necessary. Because Radiance FN is opaque, lip injection is visible on radiographs, and patients and their dentists should be made aware of this.

Autogenous fat, dermis, and fascia can be used as tissue fillers but are beyond the scope of this article [11,12]. In addition, human cell–cultured products are available for injection. A tissue punch biopsy is

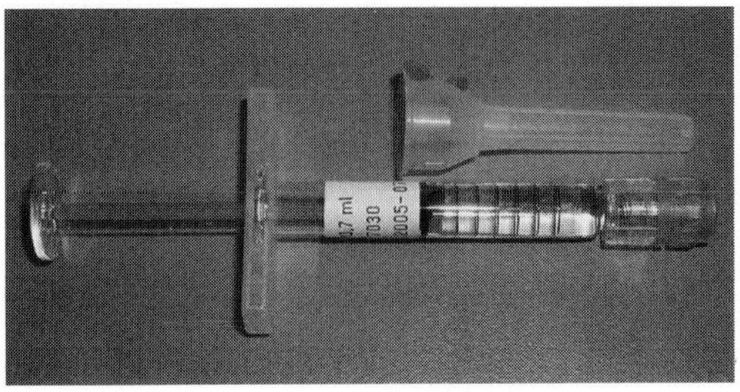

Fig. 4. The FDA approval of Restylane has created a new interest for advanced facial filler substances. Restylane comes packaged as 0.7 mL of a clear viscous gel with a supplied 30-gauge needle.

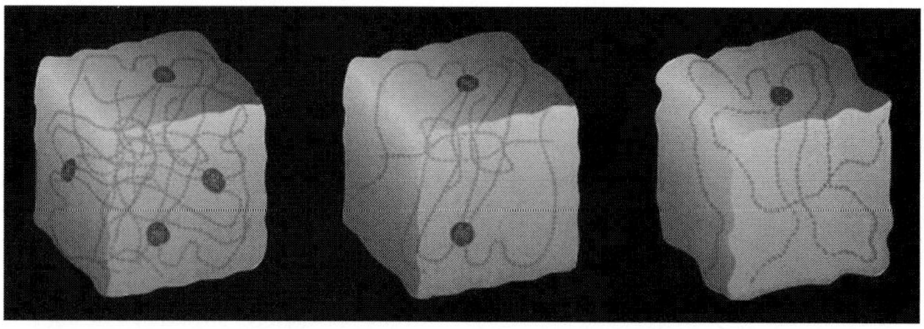

Fig. 5. Isovolemic degradation is a process of drawing water into the degrading filler molecule that maintains molecular volume in the face of degradation. The molecule degrades but draws in water, which maintains volume over time.

taken from behind the ear and cultured to derive an injectable collagen that is originally native to that patient. The process takes a number of weeks and is not seen as a major option by most cosmetic surgeons. Finally, a plethora of new products that have been used in other countries are "knocking at the doors"of the FDA. New Fill (Sculptra) (lactic acid; Advantis Pharmaceuticals, Bridgewater, NJ), Juvederm (nonanimal hyaluronic acid gel; Euromedical Systems Limited, Nottingham, UK), Artecoll and Artefill (methylmethacrylate microspheres in a hyaluronic acid vehicle; Artes Medical, San Diego, California) are just a few of the products for which approval is being sought in the United States. On the surface, some of the products that boast permanence seem appealing, but permanent fillers can lead to permanent complications. The long-term success of these products remains to be seen. Silicone has seen resurgence as a filler option but past misadventures could pose significant medicolegal problems.

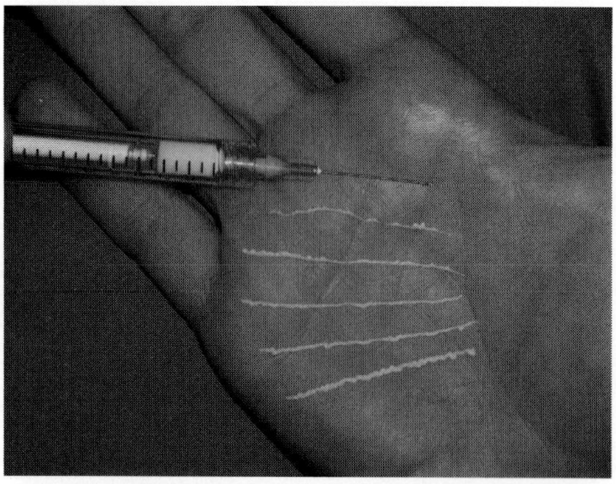

Fig. 6. Radiance FN is a hydroxyapatite paste that is opaque clinically and radiographically.

Injectable fillers: treatment considerations

Currently in the author's practice, the injection of various lip fillers is a daily occurrence. The default filler used is Restylane; however, many patients present with a specific request for a filler that they desire. Due to this patient preference, the author also injects Cosmoplast, Cosmoderm, Radiance FN, and Hyaluron. The most common requested site is the lips, followed by the nasolabial folds, the perioral region, cheek wrinkles, and "crow's feet" wrinkles. Due to the marketing hype, some patients confuse fillers with Botox. In addition, some patients desire massive rhytid injection, but because they have such a large amount of wrinkling, this would not be practical. These patients are informed that they would be better treated with lifting or resurfacing procedures. In theory, fillers can be injected anywhere on the face; however, blindness has been reported with the periorbital injection of Zyplast and fat due to intravascular injection [13–15]. This rare but devastating complication calls attention to the care that must be exercised in this area. The surgeon should always inject very superficially, use the smallest-gauge needle possible, and never use extreme plunger pressure on the syringe.

Although the injection of fillers is simple, many problems can result in terms of patient expectations and satisfaction. The main consideration is to accurately explain what the patient can expect as a treatment result. Because many patients have been "media victims," they present with unrealistic expectations, hoping for a miracle. Showing patients a series of before and after images for specific anatomic areas is one way to provide a reasonable expectation. In addition, the injection of fillers should not be presented as a one-time procedure but as a treatment sequence to approach a result. Especially for some of the newer fillers such as Restylane that cause immediate swelling in the lips, judging the end point and symmetry can be difficult. Having the patient return in 1 to 2 weeks gives the surgeon and the patient an opportunity to critique the result and to correct any areas of underfill or asymmetry. It should also be stated that any treatment should be conservative because more filler can easily be added. When the treatment area is overfilled or uneven, however, there is not much that can be done. Also paramount to communication is who will pay for the touch up should it be necessary. There are many means to work out this scenario, but the bottom line is that it must be decided in the informed consent before treating. The question of "how much to use" frequently arises. For the novice injector or the novice patient, they may be unaware of what to expect in terms of how much area can be effectively treated with a single syringe. Again, the surgeon must be cognizant of how far a single syringe can go. When in doubt, it is prudent to pay attention to the amount left in the syringe, and when 50% is used, the other side must be treated. Failure to do this will require a second syringe to be opened and, if the patient was not expecting another $500 fee, then unpleasant discussion may follow. When in doubt, the patient should be told that a single syringe may not be adequate for the given augmentation.

Treating the lips

Every injector has his or her way of injecting fillers, but two recognized techniques are used universally. Linear threading involves inserting the needle and injection filler as a straight line while continuously moving in either a forward or backward direction (Fig. 7). This process would be analogous to placing a line of toothpaste on one's toothbrush. The other injection method is known as the serial puncture technique. This involves placing small boluses of filler with multiple punctures along the lip or wrinkle. The wrinkle is filled by deposition of the small bolus of filler along the wrinkle and requires multiple needle sticks (see Fig. 7).

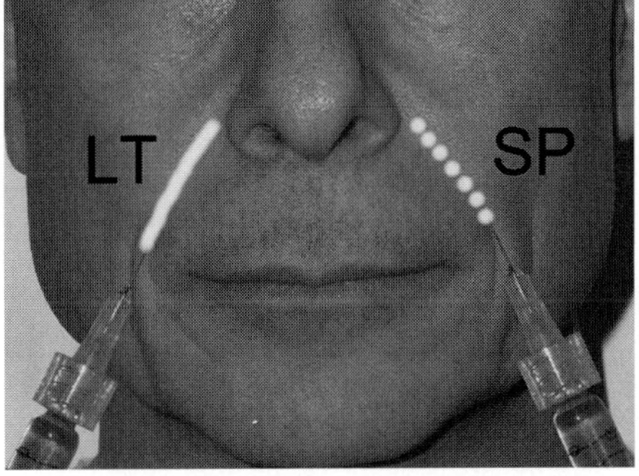

Fig. 7. Linear threading (LT) involves inserting the needle and injecting the filler in a straight line while continuously moving in either a forward or backward direction. The serial puncture (SP) technique involves placing small boluses of filler with multiple punctures along the line or wrinkle. The wrinkle is filled by placing the boluses together using multiple needle sticks.

Anesthetic considerations

Most of the new fillers do not contain any inherent local anesthesia. The author strongly recommends using local anesthetic techniques when treating the lips. Many patients can tolerate filler injections in the cutaneous areas such as the nasolabial folds or cheeks, but injecting the lips can provide significant discomfort. In addition, new, potent topical anesthetics are available. BLT cream (20% benzocaine, 6% lidocaine, and 4% tetracaine in a cream vehicle; Bayview Pharmacy, Baltimore, Maryland) is applied to the lips and vestibular mucosa. When injecting the upper lip, bilateral infraorbital blocks are administered and bilateral mental blocks are given for the lower lips [16]. Alternately, the upper and lower vestibule can be infiltrated with 3 to 4 equally spaced injections from the cuspid area on one side to the cuspid area on the other. These infiltrative injections are easier to perform than nerve blocks and usually provide the required level of anesthesia. Proper anesthesia is beneficial not only to the patient but also to the doctor; a doctor who does not inflict pain will receive positive word-of-mouth referrals.

The most common area requested is the lips. Some patients may want only a single lip (usually the upper) treated, whereas most patients desire bilabial treatment. It is important to query the patient on exactly what their expectations are. Do they want more defined lips? Do they want bigger lips? Do they want to show more vermilion? Many patients are not sophisticated enough to know exactly what they want and, therefore, rely on the surgeon to decide. This author begins conservatively with patients who have never had fillers. Generally, the white roll of Cupid's bow is injected in the intradermal or submucosal plane or both. The "M" configuration is augmented with a roll of filler extending from one oral commissure to the other. Care is used to form crisp, angular contours in the "downward legs" of the M in the area of the central lip. Most patients have this basic M pattern but, in some individuals, it must be

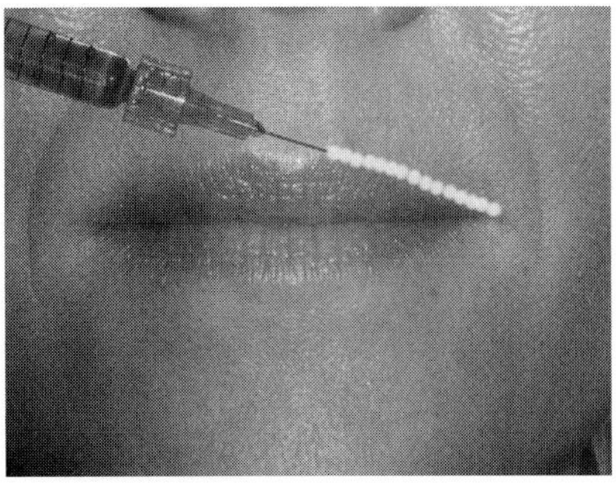

Fig. 8. The lateral lip is initially augmented from the midline to the oral commissure.

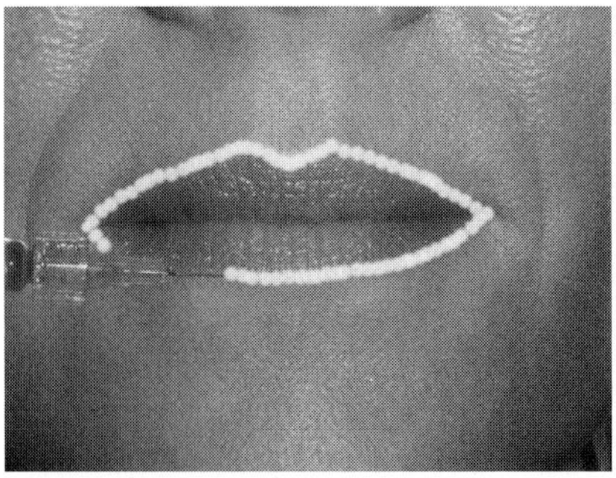

Fig. 10. The white roll is augmented to outline both lips, which generally produces subtle augmentation with increased volume and pout. Frequently, this outline also improves vertical lip rhytids by stretching the skin.

recreated. The white roll is also created in the lower lip but is more curvilinear than in the upper lip. In the average patient, the author begins lip augmentation with the upper lip and injects Restylane in the potential space just beneath the lip mucosa. The needle is inserted at the mucocutaneous junction or slightly on the mucosal side and inserted all the way to the hub. As the needle is withdrawn, the filler is evenly injected into this potential space. If the needle is in the correct plane, the filler easily flows forward and sometimes retrograde along the lip. By using the noninjecting hand to pinch the lip with the thumb and forefinger, the surgeon can contain the filler to the desired space laterally along the lip. In general, the author begins by injecting the left side of the upper lip and proceeds laterally to the commissure (Fig. 8). Next, the same procedure is performed on the right side of the lip. Finally, the descending legs of the central M configuration are injected to make sharp angles in the central upper lip (Fig. 9). It is important to be conservative in this area or the patient will have a "ducky" look in the lateral view.

The lower lip is injected in a similar manner but without sharp angles (Fig. 10). The filler is injected in the potential space just beneath the mucosa across the entire lower lip.

Sometimes, a single syringe is sufficient to outline the upper lip but not the entire lower lip. In this case, injecting only the middle third of the lip provides a nice central augmentation, producing a "shine" of light reflex when wearing lipstick or lip gloss that is appreciated by most women. Some patients benefit from this central augmentation only, whereas others require augmentation across the entire lip.

Outlining the white roll around both lips is enough cosmetic enhancement for many patients. Some patients may desire more vermilion volume and want bigger lips as opposed to simply more-defined lips. The author accommodates these patients by injecting more filler in each lip but in a slightly different manner. Instead of injecting at the vermilion/cutaneous junction, the needle is inserted several millimeters below the cutaneous margin and well into the vermilion. Depending on the desired area to be augmented, the needle is sometimes positioned at the wet/dry line. Again, the needle is inserted to the hub

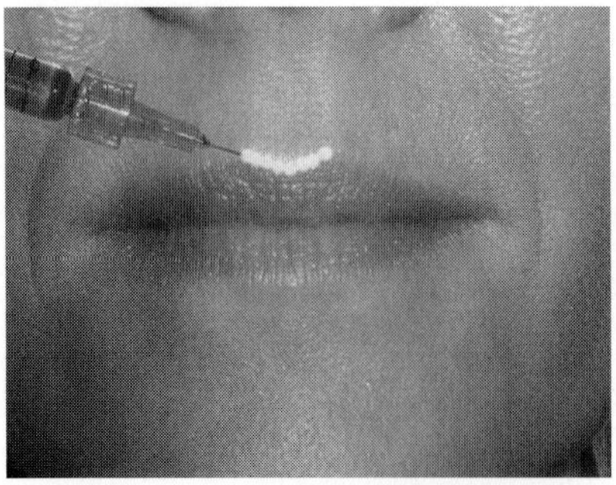

Fig. 9. The next step is to augment the M configuration of the upper lip. Recreating this angular configuration increases the esthetics of the lip.

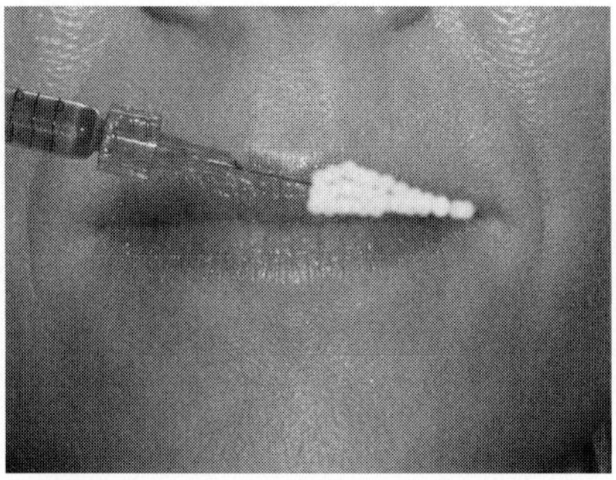

Fig. 11. After the white roll is outlined, the vermilion area can further be augmented if esthetics dictate or the patient desires.

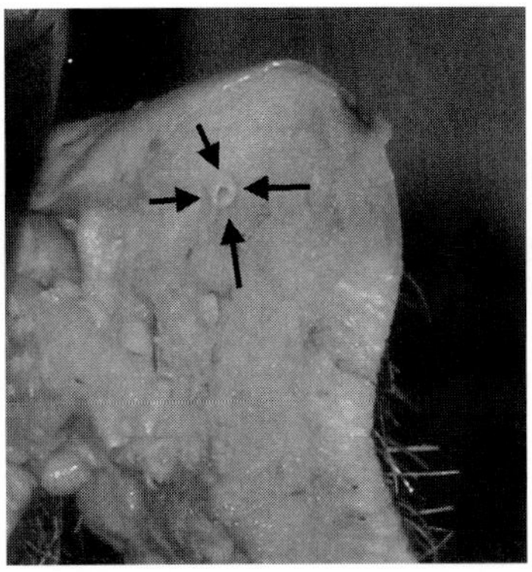

Fig. 12. The labial artery (*arrows*) usually traverses the upper, posterior one third of the lower lip at the level of the incisal edge of the lower anterior teeth.

and slowly withdrawn while continuous, steady injection is performed. In this area, the goal is to spread a thin, flat layer to plump the vermilion (Fig. 11). The needle can also be placed deeper into the lip when greater volume is required.

Other than inadvertent vascular puncture with resultant hematoma, there is no danger in deeper injections in the lip (this obviously excludes intravascular injection, which could cause lip necrosis). Fig. 12 shows the relationship of the labial artery to the lip. Notice that the artery lies in the posterior one third of the lip at about the level of the incisal edge of the anterior teeth [17]. This level also corresponds with the vermilion/cutaneous junction on the facial surface of the lip.

Augmenting the lips by using the techniques of outlining the white roll and augmenting the vermilion may be too large of an augmentation for a novice surgeon or a first-time patient. For the inexperienced injector or a first-time augmentation, the author recommends doing only the white roll outline technique and re-evaluating the patient's satisfaction in a week or two. At that follow-up appointment, the secondary vermilion injection may be accomplished. The main reason for this dual-treatment sequence is to prevent overaugmentation of the lips that make take many months to resolve. With experience, the surgeon and the patient can gauge how much and what areas can be done simultaneously.

Injecting oral commissures

Perioral aging frequently causes depressed triangular areas at each oral commissure. Not only are these depressions unaesthetic but they also cause a "down-turned" smile. This area must be addressed when treating the lips. One problem is that these depressions represent the convergence of multiple tissue planes, and a significant amount of filler can be injected here without significant augmentation. In the author's experience, it takes at least an entire syringe (one half on each side) to make a difference on the oral commissures. Also, if the filler is injected deep, it fails to make much of a difference on the augmentation; it just seems to disappear into the deeper tissues. To combat this situation, some filler is injected deeper to create a base and then the remainder is injected more superficially in the dermis to plump out the depression. In some patients, this area does not improve significantly with fillers and presents a challenge for cosmetic improvement. Face-lift and laser resurfacing can also assist this area.

An encapsulation of the previous augmentation strategy needs to be underlined by the fact that facial augmentation with fillers is a form of artistry and, therefore, no hard rules exist on what is the correct way to do it and what the final desired result should be. What is important is that the patients are happy with the result. By following the presented basic augmentation techniques of white roll outline and vermilion fill, most practitioners can deliver pleasing results to their patients. The true form of artistry comes in to effect with various subtleties, among them, augmentation of the philtral columns. In a well-defined lip, the philtrum is a depression bordered on each side by triangular columns, with the apex at the ala and the base at the vermilion. The columns border an almond-shaped depression, which is the philtrum. Even the most-experienced injectors oftentimes fail to augment this area. Some patients have a somewhat defined philtral area and by augmenting what they have, the result can be very pleasing. In other patients, virtually no philtral column definition exists

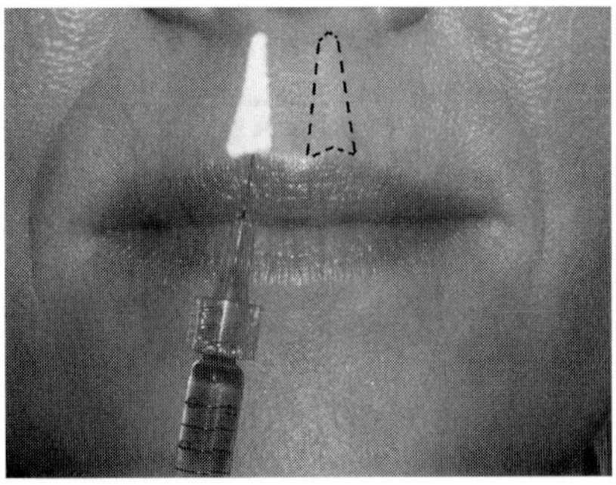

Fig. 13. The philtral columns are injected in a reverse taper from the narrower alar base to the broader vermilion border.

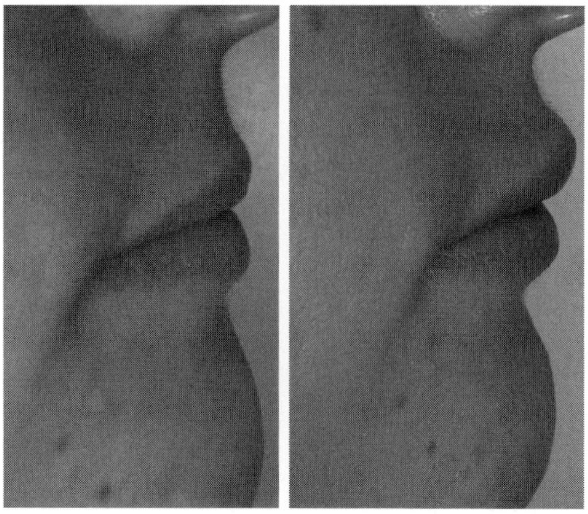

Fig. 14. Lateral view of before (*left image*) and 2 weeks after (*right image*) Restylane injection of the upper and lower lips.

and in these patients, the anatomy must be created. To enhance the philtral columns, the needle is inserted at the vermilion/cutaneous junction in the intradermal plane and directed all the way to the base of the ala. The skin is then pinched with the noninjecting hand in a means to create a triangle. Less filler is injected near the alar base, with more filler injected toward the vermilion border (Fig. 13). By pinching the skin with the noninjecting hand, the injected filler can be formed into the specific shape.

Figs. 14 and 15 show lip augmentation with Restylane.

Augmenting wrinkles, lines, and folds

In addition to structural augmentation of the lips, injectable fillers are used to plump lines, folds, and wrinkles. As mentioned earlier, this process is practical for any given wrinkle, but some patients may

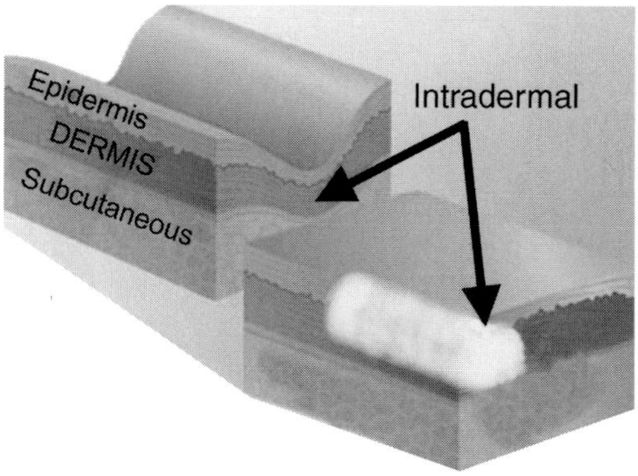

Fig. 16. Most fillers are injected in the intradermal plane.

present with severe rhytidosis and think that hundreds of wrinkles may be treated. Again, these patients must be educated to understand that they are better candidates for rhytidectomy or skin resurfacing. Patients with many wrinkles can be candidates for injectable fillers, however, so long as they understand that selected wrinkles, lines, or folds can be treated.

When injecting the facial skin, most fillers are placed intradermally (Fig. 16). One exception may be Radiance FN, which the author recommends placing somewhat deeper. Because Radiance FN is white and can lump easier than other fillers, using the deep dermis or even the subcutaneous plane is desirable. At the time of this article's publication, Restylane is the only nonanimal hyaluronic acid filler with FDA approval. Medicis offers several other fillers that are available in other countries. Perlane is similar to Restylane but has a larger particle size and is for deep dermal injection. The indication for this product is similar to Restylane, but due to the larger particle size, it must be injected deeper. Restylane Fine Line is another Medicis product. This product has a smaller particle size and is designed for more superficial dermal injection. Fine lines around the lip and

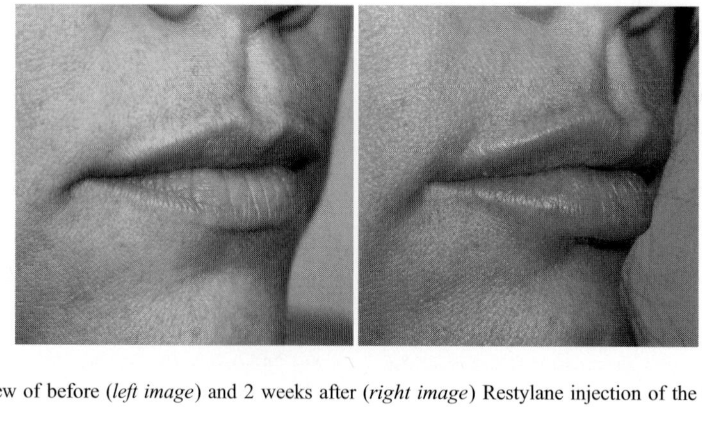

Fig. 15. Oblique view of before (*left image*) and 2 weeks after (*right image*) Restylane injection of the upper and lower lips.

crow's feet areas are common indications. This product corresponds to Cosmoderm, which has a smaller particle size than Cosmoplast. These products are human collagen derivatives. With the many choices of filler types and particle sizes, it is not uncommon for some practitioners to layer different types of fillers to achieve a desired result. Some practitioners may initially inject Perlane deep in the lip or fold and then inject Restylane more superficially. The same technique can be used with Cosmoplast injected deeply and Cosmoderm injected more superficially. The United States' experience is likely to mirror that of other countries, which means that many types and choices of fillers are likely to become available in the next several years.

Injecting perioral rhytids

Among the features of aging that disturb female patients the most are perioral vertical rhytids. These wrinkles are also called lipstick lines because applied lipstick tends to flow through these lines and enhance these telltale signs of aging. When patients present for the treatment of perioral rhytids, they are informed that there are several means to treat these wrinkles. This author oftentimes treats the lip as mentioned earlier by recreating (or augmenting) the white roll around the upper and lower lips. In many cases, simply by doing this, the skin is stretched and many perioral lines are improved. More substantial perioral lines need to be individually injected in the intradermal plane. Restylane Fine Line or Cosmoderm are fillers specifically formulated for superficial rhytids.

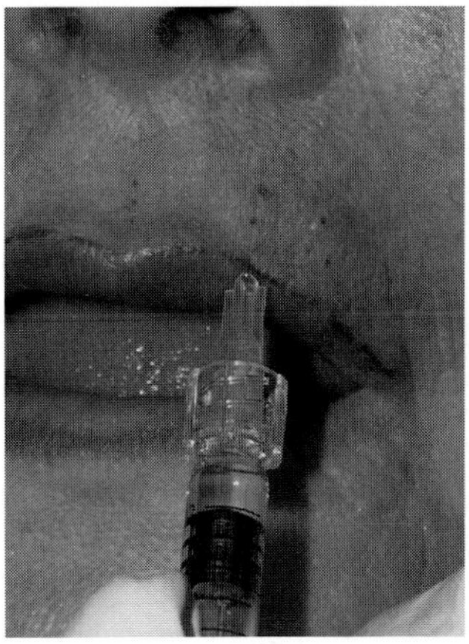

Fig. 17. Perioral rhytids may improve with circumferential white roll augmentation, but may also be treated individually by intradermal injection.

The injection technique is performed by injecting the finer particle–sized products more superficially into the dermis. For these wrinkles, the author places the needle at the vermilion/cutaneous border in the superficial dermal plane and inserts the needle to the hub. The needle is then withdrawn while injecting (linear threading technique). This technique is repeated on neighboring wrinkles (Fig. 17). A general concept is that fillers do not last as long in areas of increased movement (such as the lips) as in areas of decreased movement (such as malar augmentation).

Injecting the nasolabial folds

This area is high on many patients' list for filler injection. It is noteworthy to mention that patients with extremely deep nasolabial folds are not the best candidates because they are likely to be disappointed with the result. Many patients desire total ablation of their nasolabial folds and pull back their skin to show their perceived result. It must be explained to the patient that injecting a filler substance does not make these folds go away; furthermore, an adult patient would look unnatural without any nasolabial fold. It is further explained that the purpose of injecting the nasolabial fold is to blunt the area to mitigate the severity. Discussion also needs to be presented about the number of syringes required to receive the result. Many patients read about fillers in a woman's magazine and present to "test the waters." They oftentimes only desire to invest in a single syringe of filler but wish to have both nasolabial folds treated, which presents a treatment dilemma. A single syringe is usually not enough to make much difference bilaterally, especially in advanced aging. By granting the patient's wish of a single syringe, the result is likely to be minimal. If this is the case, the patient will be unhappy and it may reflect on their perception of the doctor. The author explains to the patient that although a single syringe can be used, it is not likely to make a significant difference bilaterally. Some of the author's best results have entailed using a single syringe in each fold and having the patient return several weeks later to repeat injection with another two syringes. This treatment is obviously an expensive one, but to deliver substantial results, substantial amounts of filler are required in this area, unless the patient has minimal folds.

Injecting the nasolabial folds requires practice, and there are a number of caveats involved. The patient should never have the nasolabial fold area injected while in the supine or recumbent position because the gravitational effects distort the nasolabial

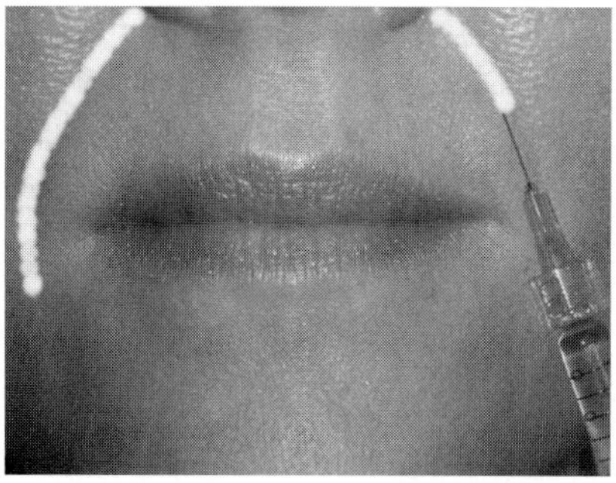

Fig. 18. The nasolabial folds are augmented by filling the valley of the fold with injection slightly medial to the fold. The linear threading technique and serial puncture technique can be used singularly or together to achieve the desired clinical result.

area. The patient should always be seated upright. The most important pitfall to avoid is having the filler migrate laterally in the fold. This situation can happen easily and, if it occurs, can make the nasolabial fold larger because the filler creates a bigger ridge on the lateral cheek. To prevent this problem, it is imperative to observe where the filler is flowing and to err on the medial side of the fold. By staying medial, the filler usually remains in the valley of the fold and, thus, causes the desired blunting effect (Fig. 18).

This area is one where the author uses the linear threading and serial puncture technique concomitantly. The syringe is inserted in the intradermal plane to the hub and filler is injected as the syringe is withdrawn (linear threading). When this process is not sufficient to produce enough augmentation, small boluses of filler are injected along the fold (serial puncture technique). By alternating these two techniques, the fold can be augmented naturally. It should be mentioned that if many punctures are used over a given area, the filler can leak out on injection. If this occurs in multiple areas along the fold, the session is stopped and continued in 1 to 2 weeks. For significant nasolabial augmentation, it is a good idea to make it a multiple-event procedure. More accurate augmentation can be performed over two appointments. Fig. 19 shows nasolabial fold augmentation with Radiance FN.

The technique for injecting other facial lines and wrinkles is very similar. These injections are intradermal and can be performed by linear threading, serial puncture, or a combination of both. Common areas to inject include lateral canthal (crow's feet) wrinkles, glabelar wrinkles, frontalis wrinkles, mentolabial fold wrinkles, and cheek wrinkles.

Complications

Complications seen with injectable fillers are usually minor [18–23], although as mentioned earlier, blindness has been reported after injecting near the periorbita. The main complications seen with fillers include the following:

Intravascular injection
Tissue necrosis
Bruising
Excessive swelling
Hematoma
Bruising
Needle tracks
Asymmetry
Overfill
Underfill
Contour irregularities (lumpiness)
Material visible through skin (injection too superficial)
Herpes simplex activation

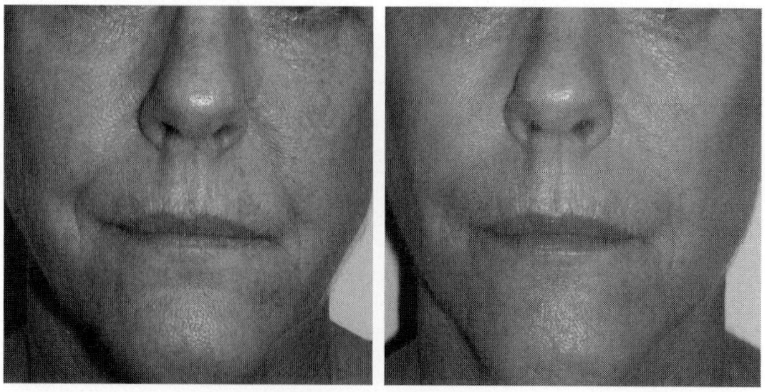

Fig. 19. Before (*left image*) and 3 weeks after (*right image*) augmentation of nasolabial folds with Radiance FN.

Most of these complications represent minor or transient problems that self-correct or improve. Intravascular injection can cause tissue necrosis. Necrosis can also be seen from vascular congestion from injections that compromise the dermal plexus. Sometimes, tissue blanching can be seen while injecting, which is usually transient, but in some cases, vascular refill does not happen and areas of tissue slough are seen. This situation can be prevented by paying attention to the plane of injection and not overinjecting or injecting with excessive pressure to produce blanching.

Hematoma and bruising are very disconcerting to the patient and can effect the reputation of the surgeon. Patients who take drugs, medications, or herbal preparations such as gingko, garlic, ginseng, or St. John's wort should stop these medications 2 weeks before filler injection. Most swelling resolves within 24 to 48 hours Occasionally, excessive swelling is seen after filler injection, especially in the lips. These patients usually respond well to heat, elevation, and tapering steroid treatment. Patients should be forewarned that hyaluronic acid products produce more swelling than collagen products.

As with any procedure, a sound preoperative informed consent can mitigate potential post-treatment problems. The consent should not only cover the main complications but also address the need for follow-up treatments and specify how touch-up injections will be handled financially (many patients expect the surgeon to absorb the cost; to avoid miscommunication, this topic should specifically be addressed). The author frequently provides touch-up injections at a significantly reduced rate, especially when the cause is due to a problem on the surgeon's part, such as asymmetry. Of all caveats, being a conservative injector and having the patient return for follow-up evaluation is perhaps the most important. It is important to not overfill treated areas because the surgeon can always add more filler; after it is injected, it persists for months (Fig. 20).

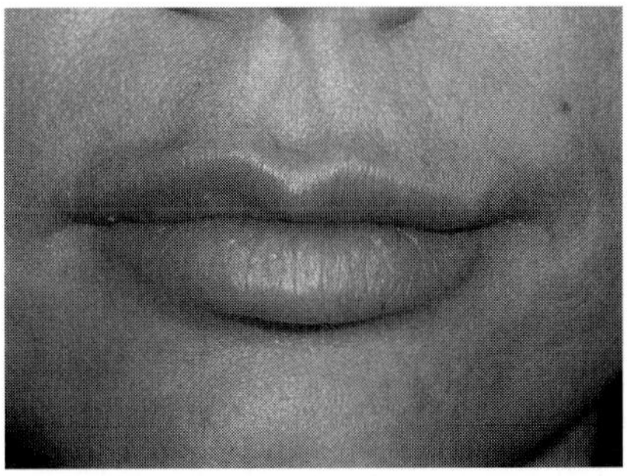

Fig. 20. This image illustrates post-treatment asymmetry. Notice that the patient's left side of the upper lip is significantly underfilled compared with the right side. The patient was brought back for touch-up and required 0.3 mL of Restylane to balance the symmetry.

It also is important to take a series of preoperative photographs of the frontal, oblique, and lateral views of the area to be treated. This record can assist the surgeon and the patient in many ways. Frequently, patients forget what their lips looked like before injection and can be overly critical of the result. Referring to the preoperative photographs can be helpful in this circumstance. In addition, these images can be used for marketing or, more important, to show prospective patients anticipated results.

Summary

Cosmetic facial surgery is an integral part of the specialty of oral and maxillofacial surgery, and injectable facial fillers fit well into the armamentarium of the contemporary oral and maxillofacial surgeon. These procedures are generally simple to learn, provide high patient and doctor satisfaction, and produce few complications.

References

[1] Klein AW. Paraffinomas of the scalp. Arch Dermatol 1985;121:382–5.
[2] Palkhivala A. Injected silicone risks. Dermatology Times June 2003;69.
[3] Keefe J, Wauk L, Chu S, et al. Clinical use of injectable bovine collagen: a decade of experience. Clin Mater 1992;9(3–4):155–62.
[4] Olenius M. The first clinical study using a new biodegradable implant for the treatment of lips, wrinkles, and folds. Aesthetic Plast Surg 1998;22(2):97–101.
[5] Narins RS, Brandt F, Leyden J, et al. A randomized, double-blind, multicenter comparison of the efficacy and tolerability of Restylane versus Zyplast for the correction of nasolabial folds. Dermatol Surg 2003; 29(6):588–95.
[6] Lemperle G, Morhenn VV, Charrier U. Human histology and persistence of various injectable filler substances for soft tissue augmentation. Aesthetic Plast Surg 2003;27(5):354–66.
[7] Q Med, Inc., Information brochure. Uppsalla, Sweden.
[8] Duranti F, Salti G, Bovani B, et al. Injectable hyaluronic acid gel for soft tissue augmentation. A clinical and histological study. Dermatol Surg 1998;24(12): 1317–25.

[9] Bosniak S, Cantisano-Zilkha M. Restylane and Perlane: a review of safety and effectiveness. Operat Techn Oculoplast Orbital Reconstr Surg 2003;4(7): 491–4.
[10] Sklar JA, Soren M, White MD. Radiance FN: a new soft tissue filler. Derm Surg 2004;30(5):764–8.
[11] Niamtu J. Clinical technique for fat transfer. Cosmetic facial surgery. Oral Maxillofacial Surg Clin N Am 2000;12(4):641–7.
[12] Niamtu J. Fat transfer gun used as a precision injection device for injectable soft tissue fillers. J Oral Maxillofac Surg 2002;60(7):838–9.
[13] Teimourian B. Blindness following fat injections. Plast Reconstr Surg 1988;82(2):361.
[14] Castillo GD. Management of blindness in the practice of cosmetic surgery. Otolaryngol Head Neck Surg 1989;100(6):559–62.
[15] Egido JA, Arroyo R, Marcos A, et al. Middle cerebral artery embolism and unilateral visual loss after autologous fat injection into the glabellar area. Stroke 1993; 24:615–6.
[16] Niamtu J. Local anesthetic blocks of the head and neck for cosmetic facial surgery. Part I. A review of basic sensory neuroanatomy. Cosmet Dermatol 2004;17: 515–22.
[17] Larrabee WF, Makielski KH, editors. Surgical anatomy of the face. New York, NY: Raven Press; 1993.
[18] Hanke CW, Higley HR, Jolivette DM, et al. Abscess formation and local necrosis after treatment with Zyderm or Zyplast collagen implant. J Am Acad Dermatol 1991;25:319–26.
[19] Friedman PM, Mafong EA, Kauvar AN, et al. Safety data of injectable nonanimal stabilized hyaluronic acid gel for soft tissue augmentation. Dermatol Surg 2002; 28(6):491–4.
[20] Lowe NJ, Maxwell CA, Lowe P, et al. Hyaluronic acid skin fillers: adverse reactions and skin testing. J Am Acad Dermatol 2001;45(6):930–3.
[21] Lupton JR, Alster TS. Cutaneous hypersensitivity reaction to injectable hyaluronic acid gel. Dermatol Surg 2000;26:135–7.
[22] Fernandez-Acenero MJ, Zamora E, Borbujo J. Granulomatous foreign body reaction against hyaluronic acid: report of a case after lip augmentation. Dermatol Surg 2003;29(12):1225–6.
[23] Honig JF, Brink U, Korabiowska M. Severe granulomatous allergic tissue reaction after hyaluronic acid injection in the treatment of facial lines and its surgical correction. J Craniofac Surg 2003;14(2): 197–200.

ELSEVIER
SAUNDERS

Oral Maxillofacial Surg Clin N Am 17 (2005) 29 – 39

ORAL AND
MAXILLOFACIAL
SURGERY CLINICS
of North America

Advanta Facial Implants

Joseph Niamtu III, DMD

Oral/Maxillofacial and Cosmetic Facial Surgery, 10230 Cherokee Road, Richmond, VA 23235, USA

There has been a huge increase in patients seeking cosmetic surgery. Many factors are driving this increase. Foremost is the fact that the baby boomers are turning 50 years old at an alarming rate of one every 8 seconds. This generation is the one that "would not age" and the one that basked in the sun with an admixture of baby oil to develop a savage tan. Other factors affecting this increase include the fact that more specialties are performing cosmetic facial surgery. The past 20 years have brought about an increase in cosmetic procedures in dermatology; oral and maxillofacial surgery; ophthalmology; oculoplastic surgery; ear, nose, and throat; and other specialties. In addition, changes of great magnitude have occurred in the health care system. Many surgeons have transitioned from a hospital-based practice to an office/surgery center environment. This environment makes the surgical experience easier, less expensive, and more personal, with increased anonymity. Finally, technologic increases in anesthesia, equipment, and procedures have made it easier than ever to have cosmetic surgery. The media (including television reality shows) and individual physician marketing also have heightened the presence of cosmetic surgery. In short, this is a great time in history for cosmetic surgery. These factors have also led to a request for minimally invasive cosmetic procedures [1]. Today's patients do not want to miss work or play and desire "wash and wear" surgical procedures. Botulinum toxin type A (Botox), Restylane, nonablative lasers, and facial implants are examples of minimally invasive cosmetic facial surgery.

E-mail address: niamtu@niamtu.com

Facial implants have been used for many years and have included a plethora of materials. Contemporary choices for fillers include fat, expanded polytetrafluoroethylene ([ePTFE] Gore-Tex; W.L. Gore Co., Flagstaff, Arizona), Silicone, Silastic, polyethylene, bovine collagen, human collagen, hydroxyapatite, acrylic microspheres, lactic acid, dermis, fascia, and others [2]. The remainder of this article addresses a specific brand of facial implant: Advanta (Atrium Medical, Hudson, New Hampshire).

Gore-Tex was developed by the W.L. Gore Company and has been used successfully for bioimplantation for 30 years [3–38]. ePTFE is basically Teflon, which is processed with a microporous configuration. This material has many unique properties. It is extremely biocompatible and does not form thick encapsulation as some materials do. For this reason, it is tissue friendly and can easily be removed if necessary. I began using Gore-Tex for facial implantation in 1996 and used it in multiple applications. I have placed over 100 Gore-Tex chin implants and this remains my material of choice for chin implantation. I also have used Gore-Tex cheek implants and these have worked well. I always anchor these implants with microfixation screws, which I believe has increased my success rate.

Despite having excellent experience with Gore-Tex chin and cheek implants, I have experienced less than satisfactory results with Gore-Tex soft tissue implants. In all fairness, any surgeon must factor in their learning curve and specific skill when judging any implant. I believe that techniques for implantation are in line with the standard of care and that most of the problems I experienced with Gore-Tex soft tissue implants were a result of the implant or level of placement. I have placed over 20 Gore-Tex multistrand implants in nasolabial folds over the past

1042-3699/05/$ – see front matter
doi:10.1016/j.coms.2004.09.007

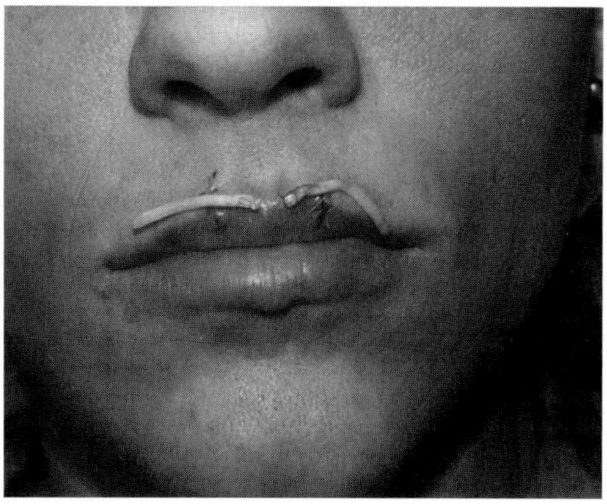

Fig. 1. Deformed, hardened, and contracted ePTFE implants removed 6 months after placement in the white roll area of the lip.

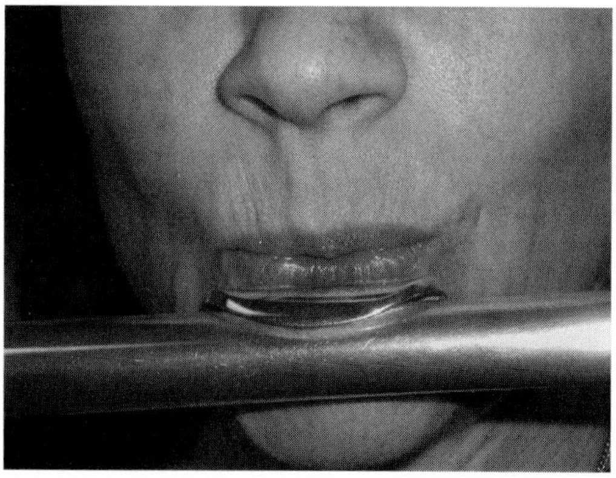

Fig. 3. This patient requested removal of her upper-lip implant due to the fact that it impeded her flute playing.

8 years. None of these have failed, and most patients are happy with their result. The biggest complaint is that the implants are palpable. I also have placed these multistrand implants in the lips and was not happy because they seemed to harden over time, becoming more visible and palpable. My biggest problems, however, have resulted from placing the small single-strand Gore-Tex implants superficially in the lip to reconstruct the "white roll." I placed many of these implants by threading the implant with a trocar from one commissure to the other. Initially, the patients and I were very happy with the result. Over several months, many of these patients presented with hardened and contracted implants that showed distortion of the lip and became significantly more visible and palpable. After removing these implants (which is an easy task), the implants were yellowed and contracted and frequently convoluted (Fig. 1).

Again, all clinicians must be fair when being critical of a product or technique. It may well be that these implants do not work when placed superficially in an area of significant movement. Although I still have patients with these implants who are pleased, I removed enough so that I ceased placing them. Due to this rate of implant removal, I took a several-year hiatus from placing lip implants (with the exception of injectable fillers).

While attending a cosmetic symposium sponsored by the American Academy of Cosmetic Surgery, I had a conversation with my friend and distinguished cosmetic dermatologist Dr. William Hanke. I related my previous problems with ePTFE implants in the lips and he told me of his experience with a new type of ePTFE facial implant called Advanta. He believed

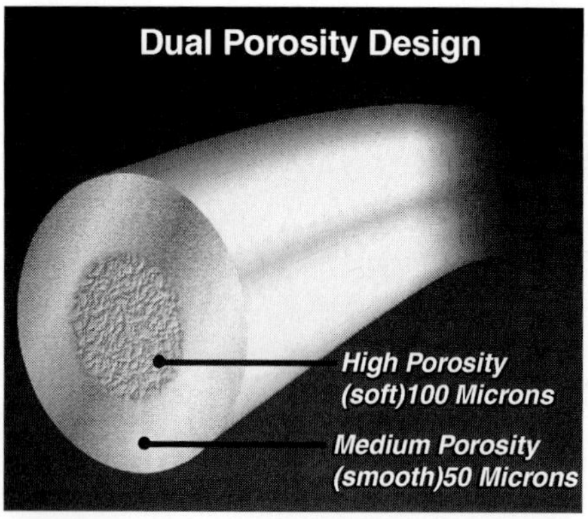

Fig. 2. The unique structure of the Advanta^{TM} dual-porosity ePTFE facial implant. (Courtesy of Atrium Medical Corporation, Hudson, NH.)

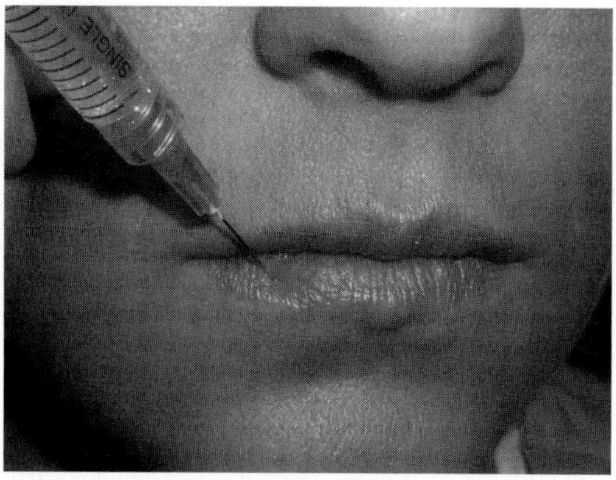

Fig. 4. Minimal infiltration across the lip vermilion and commissures is usually adequate for Advanta implant placement.

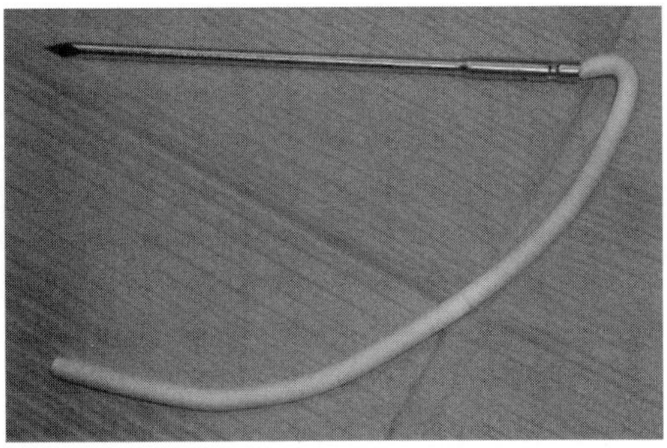

Fig. 5. It is necessary to measure the prospective implant with the mouth wide open. The error in this patient is 29% if the implant were measured in the closed-mouth position.

that the manufacturing process of this new product was superior and my experience would change as his did. After some time, Hanke [39] and Truswell [40] published their work, which led me to push ahead with this implant.

My investigations showed that the Advanta implants were different from the Gore-Tex implants I had used previously. They felt much more silky, soft, and pliable. The manufacturer attributes this look and feel to a sintering process in which the material is heated to impart these properties. In addition, the difference in this implant is the unique dual-core construction. Advanta implants are available in round or oval configurations and have an outer, medium-porosity smooth core of 50 μm and an inner, high-porosity soft core of 100 μm (Fig. 2).

This unique configuration and manufacturing process add up to make an implant that is different from what I have experienced in the past. When patients inquire about Advanta implants, I let them handle a sample to show then what will be going into their lip. They appreciate knowing what the material looks and feels like.

Patient selection

Most any healthy patient who desires lip augmentation is a candidate for Advanta implants. I believe that any lip implant should be used with caution (or not at all) in patients who play woodwind instruments, who have oral habits such as nail biting or pencil biting, or who continually fidget with their lips (Fig. 3).

Also, patients who are emotionally resistant to foreign-body implantation are not candidates. This seems obvious, but some patients will express "not liking" an implant yet will consent to the procedure. They may later come to "fear" the foreign material and request removal. Many patients will present for lip augmentation on a whim after reading an article or seeing a movie star with pretty lips. An astute surgeon must "feel out" these patients to see whether they are appropriate candidates for such a procedure. One great thing about Advanta lip implants is that they take 10 minutes to put in and 10 minutes to remove, so the procedure is effectively reversible. I believe that treating a prospective patient with a temporary injectable filler is sometimes a good idea to see how they like having fuller lips. Some patients will specifically request lip implants for several reasons. First, they are permanent. Second, they are cost effective because in my practice, the fee for a single lip implant is $1000 and the fee for a syringe of injectable filler is $440. Because the filler must be repeated, the implant is more cost effective. Finally, some patients are "needle phobic" and would rather undergo a single surgical procedure instead of multiple needle procedures.

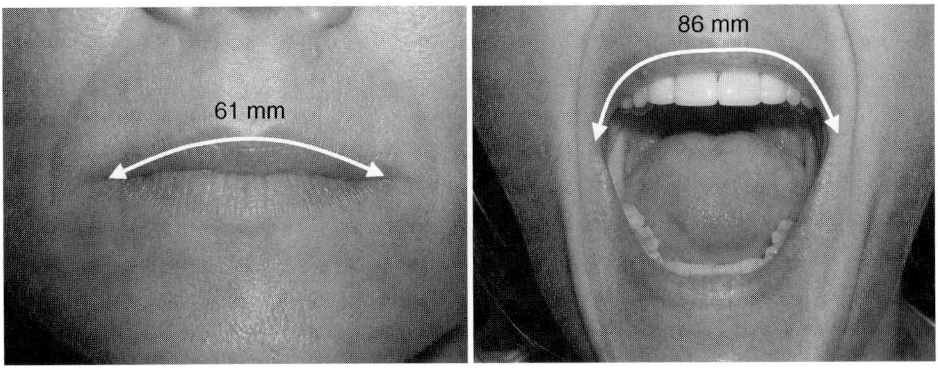

Fig. 6. The 4.0-mm round Advanta facial implant on a swaged trocar.

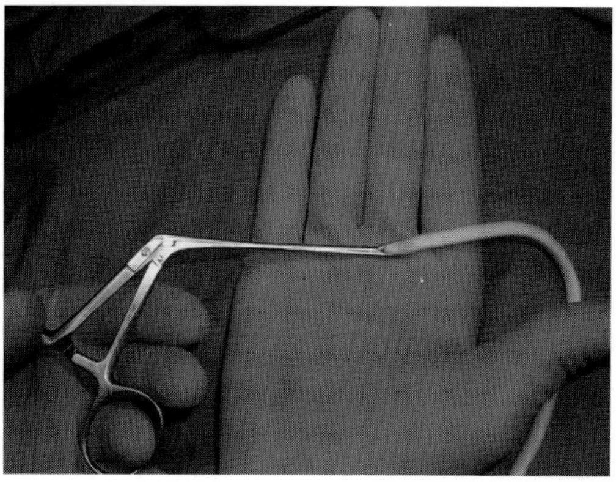

Fig. 7. A tendon passer with teeth and a tapered beak can be used to pass the implant.

It is important to let patients know in advance that they will be able to feel the implant (just like breast implants), but normal function such as smiling, kissing, and so forth is normally not affected. Patients also must realize that the implant may be visible in some extreme animations such as stretching the lips over the teeth. I remain impressed by how little these implants effect function.

Surgical placement

Placing Advanta implants in the lip is a simple procedure, but strict adherence to several principles must be maintained. Generally, I place these implants with local anesthesia. I use topical anesthesia on the mucosa, followed by local anesthetic infiltration across the lip from commissure to commissure. It does not require much anesthetic solution to render the lips insensate, and it is important to not overinject

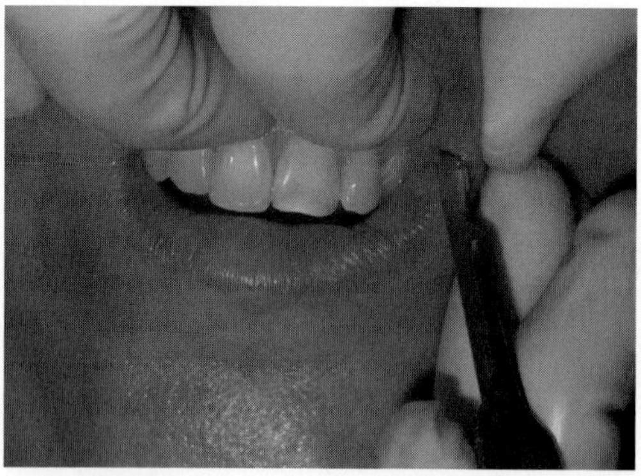

Fig. 8. The incision is made several millimeters medial to each oral commissure.

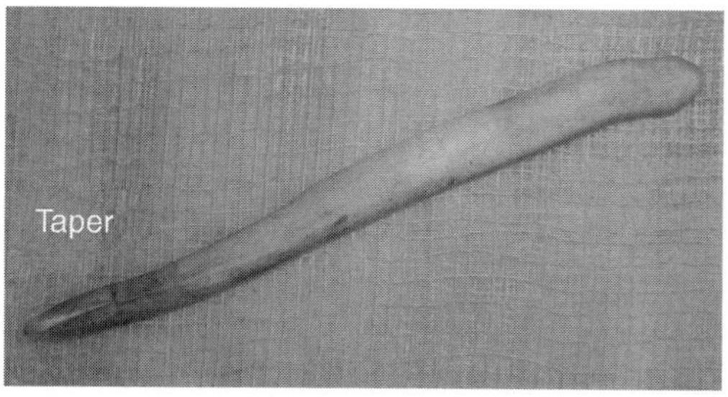

Fig. 9. Attempting to pull the implant through an incision that is not generous enough will result in a tapering of the implant.

the lip because the anesthetic volume will distort the lip and possibly skew the surgical judgment of placement (Fig. 4).

Most patients will request implants in both lips, but some patients will want to "test the waters" with a single implant.

Implant measurement

Like any new procedure or procedure that is new to a practitioner, a learning curve exists. The biggest pitfall in my experience is placing an implant in the lips that is too short. It is stated that the implant should be measured by placing it over the lips from one commissure to the other. Some practitioners neglect to say that the mouth should be maximally opened during the measurement or the implant will be too short (Fig. 5).

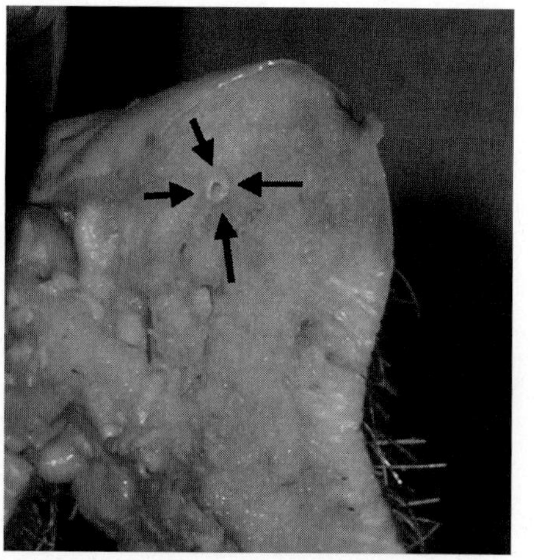

Fig. 10. The labial artery courses through the posterior one third of the lip and is usually not a problem in implant placement.

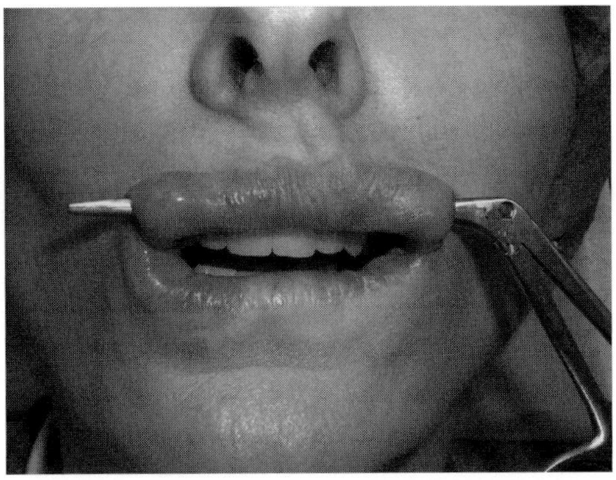

Fig. 11. The tendon passer is threaded from the entrance to the exit incision and the implant is then pulled back through the lip.

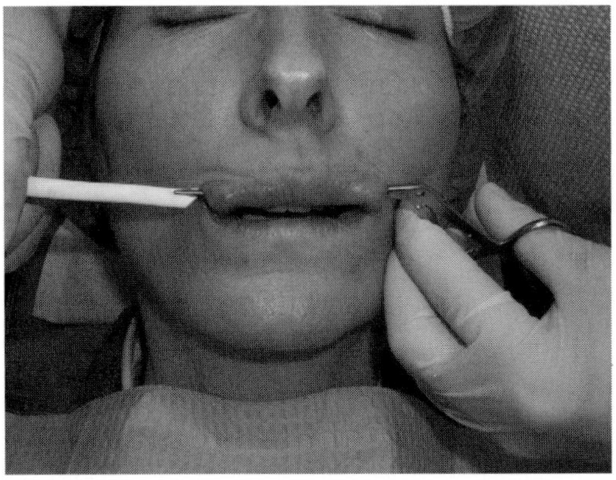

Fig. 13. The implant is grasped with the tendon passer and pulled back through the incision.

After adequate local anesthesia, I place the implant (which comes in 15-cm lengths) over the lip while the patient opens his or her mouth to the maximum opening. The implant should reach both commissures. In some patients, a single 15-cm implant can supply enough material to augment both lips, but it is a mistake to try to obtain two implants from a single strand in all patients because some patients have longer lips and the implant will fall short.

The Advanta implants for lip augmentation are available in various sizes and in round and oval configurations. I prefer the 5.0-mm round implant for most lip augmentation. In very small patients or those wanting minimal augmentation, I may elect to use a 4.0-mm implant. I initially used the oval implants but abandoned this configuration because no matter how a round implant is placed, it will remain round. An oval implant, on the other hand, may provide different contour in the same area if twisted (if the oval implant does not lay flat, one part of the lip could be more augmented than the other). At the time of this publication, only the 4.0-mm implants are available on a swaged trocar (Fig. 6). It is my hope that Atrium Medical will make a suitable trocar for the 5.0-mm implant because it assists implant placement.

The basic premise of implant placement is to make stab incisions at both commissures and to thread the implant through the lip. The implant may be pulled through the lip with multiple modalities including a passing awl and suture, a passing instrument such as a tendon passer, or an included trocar. I most frequently use a tapered tendon passer with teeth (Fig. 7).

After adequate local anesthesia, a No. 11 scalpel blade is used to make a stab incision just medial to each commissure (Fig. 8). It is important to make the length of this incision large enough to accommodate

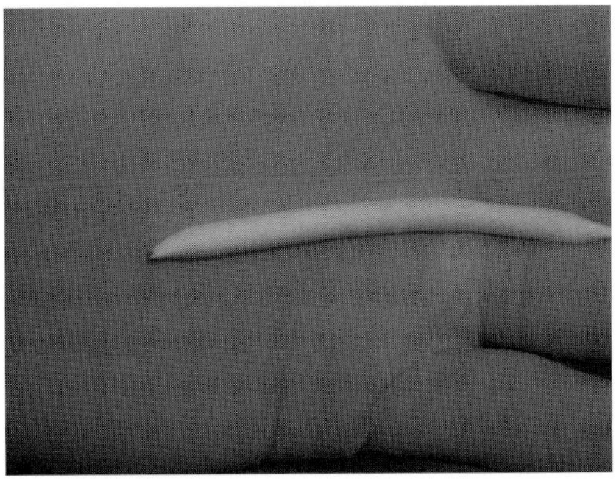

Fig. 12. The implant edges are tapered to enhance insertion and to tuck into the stab incisions.

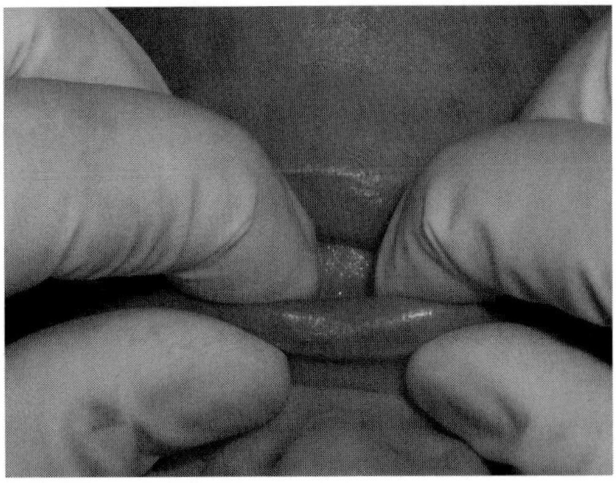

Fig. 14. After passing the implant, the lip is then stretched to fully accommodate the implant.

the implant with out distorting it. If the incision is not long enough, then the implant will exhibit ductility and will be tapered along the leading edge (Fig. 9), which will cause smaller augmentation on the leading edge and larger augmentation on the following edge. Another important principle to adhere to is the level of placement of the implant. Basically, I aim for the exact center of the lip to place the implant, which would be in a submuscular plane. If the implant is placed too superficially, then it will be visible and impede normal lip function. If the implant is placed too deeply, then the amount of augmentation is decreased and the labial artery is in jeopardy. The labial artery usually runs in the posterior one third of the lip (when viewed in cross-section) (Fig. 10) and is at the level of the anterior incisal plane in the lower lip [41].

After the stab incisions are made, the implant is threaded. I generally use a tendon passer (Byron Mentor, Byron Medical, Tucson, AZ [www.byron.com]) to thread the implant. Step 1 is to thread the implant from the entrance incision and out the exit incision (Fig. 11).

Again, it is imperative to remain in the same plane in the middle of the lip. As the tendon passer is advanced, the lip bunches. After the tendon passer is passed through the exit incision, the lip will need to be stretched to its normal length.

Passing this instrument will make a tunnel. The size of this tunnel should be just slightly smaller that the implant diameter. If the tunnel is too wide, then the implant will migrate; if too small, the implant will not lie correctly. A blunt instrument such as a knitting needle may be used to dilate the tunnel if necessary. Step 2 is to taper the edges of the implant to facilitate the threading and the position of the implant tail at the commissure (Fig. 12). Step 3 is to firmly grab the implant at the leading tapered edge and pull it through the tunnel (Fig. 13).

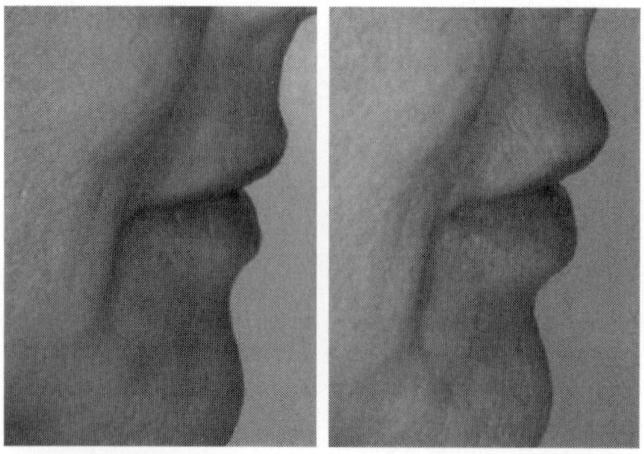

Fig. 15. A patient before (*left image*) and after (*right image*) upper- and lower-lip Advanta implants.

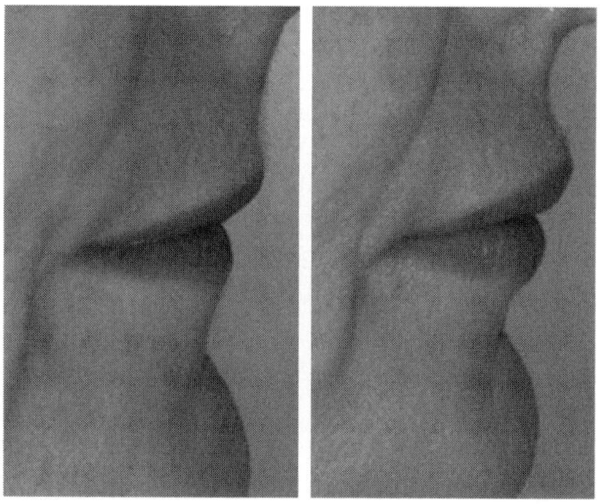

Fig. 16. A patient before (*left image*) and after (*right image*) upper- and lower-lip Advanta implants.

Having a tendon passer with teeth is helpful because it takes significant traction to pull the implant through the tunnel; it will frequently slip off the instrument if not firmly secured. Step 4 is to restrech the lip to its normal length to accommodate the implant in a natural lip position (Fig.14).

It is important to make sure that the tapered implant tails lie deep in the incision, just shy of the commissure, and do not extend outside of the incision. The final step is to close the incisions. I use 6-0 nylon suture because my experience with resorbable suture has been that the wounds dehisce.

Postoperatively, these patients are covered with cephalexin, 500 mg, every 6 hours for 5 days. The patient is asked to ice the lips for 48 hours and refrain from excessive lip function for a week. Postoperative swelling is variable. I have had patients return to work the next day and have had several patients experience severe lip swelling that took a week to

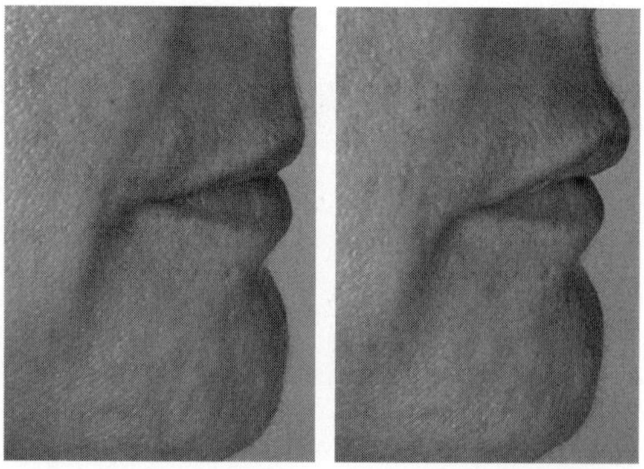

Fig. 17. A patient before (*left image*) and after (*right image*) Advanta implant in the upper lip only.

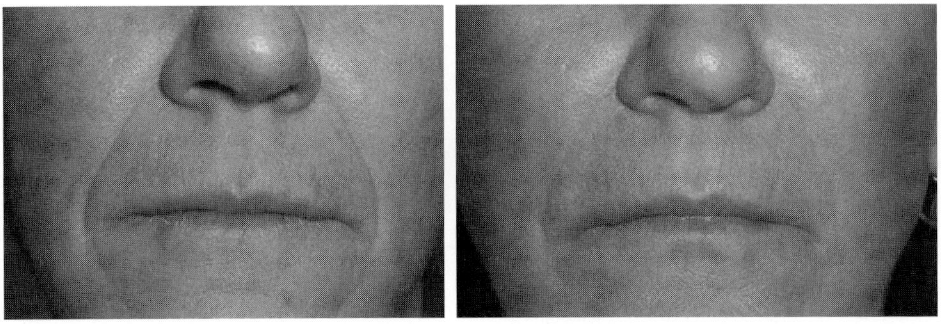

Fig. 18. This patient was treated with Advanta implants in the nasolabial folds with concomitant carbon dioxide laser resurfacing.

resolve. Preoperatively, patients must be made aware of this variable healing. Appropriate analgesics are prescribed for several days. The sutures are removed on the fifth postoperative day.

Clinical results

Figs. 15 through 18 show before and after photographs of Advanta implant lip augmentation.

Alternate site implant placement

Although I use Advanta facial implants primarily for lip augmentation, they can be used for multiple facial applications including augmentation of nasolabial folds, glabelar lines, mandibulolabial folds (drool lines), and acne scars.

To treat the nasolabial folds, the technique is similar to lip implant placement. The implant is placed in the subdermal plane. It is extremely important to make sure the implant lies within or just medial to the valley of the fold (this is a problem area for the novice surgeon). Many tissue planes come together in the nasolabial fold region and, when placing an implant (or filler) in this area, the implant can frequently displace laterally. When this happens, the implant increases the lateral portion of the nasolabial fold and makes it appear deeper. Accentuating a nasolabial fold in a patient who presented for effacement is a problem. Again, by placing the

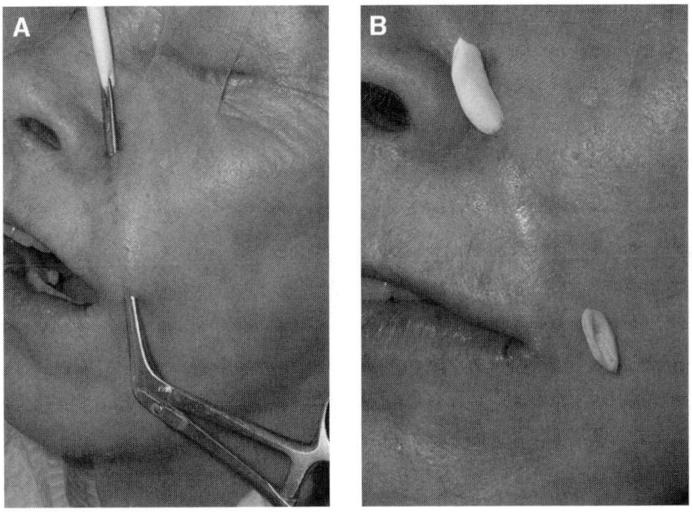

Fig. 19. (*A*) Placement of Advanta implants in the nasolabial region is similar to lip placement. (*B*) The implant will lie in the subdermal plane.

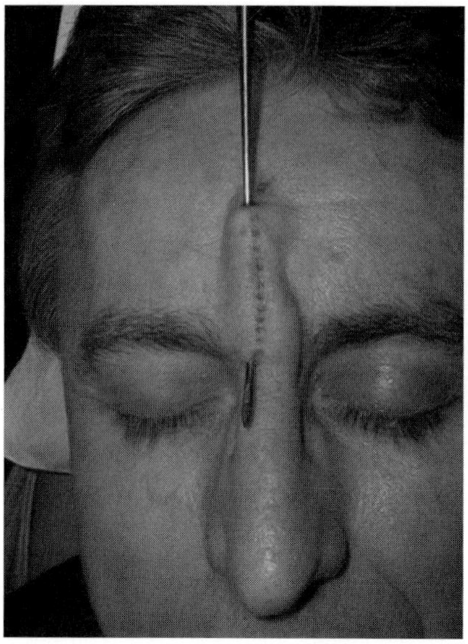

Fig. 20. A tunnel is made and a passing awl inserted to place an implant in the treatment of glabelar lines.

implant just nasally to the fold, accurate placement can be achieved. It is also important to inform the patient that an implant will not make the fold go away but will blunt the fold by decreasing the valley. It is also important for the patient to realize that the fold will be blunted in repose but still appear as a fold with animation such as smiling.

To treat the nasolabial fold, an entrance stab incision is made just inferior to the ala (although some surgeons will place the incision intranasally) and an exit stab incision is made at the inferior portion of the fold. The stab incisions are oriented to Langer's lines and are made as small as possible to accommodate the implant. These generally heal without a scar, but on occasion, I will use the carbon dioxide laser to resurface these scars to better blend them. The implant is measured (with the mouth open) and its ends are tapered. A trocar, tendon passer, or awl and suture are used to pull the implant from the superior incision through the inferior incision (Fig. 19). The skin is then stretched to passively accommodate the implant and the ends are again trimmed to just fall within the stab incisions. The incisions are then closed with 6-0 nylon suture.

Glabelar lines

Occasionally, patients will present with the complaint of deep glabelar lines that are resistant to Botox and fillers. I have treated this area successfully with ePTFE implants. In other cases, I have used ePTFE implants in combination with Botox and carbon dioxide laser resurfacing for a maximum result. The method of placement is the same as in nasolabial folds and the implant is placed in the subdermal plane. I find it helpful to also treat this area with Botox when placing a glabelar implant because I believe that the reduced movement facilitates healing. Fig. 20 shows placement of an ePTFE glabelar implant.

Fig. 21 shows before and after photographs of a patient who received an ePTFE implant, Botox, and laser resurfacing.

Mandibulolabial folds (drool lines)

Downturned corners of the mouth or depressions in this area are difficult to treat. Although I have not placed Advanta implants in this area, other

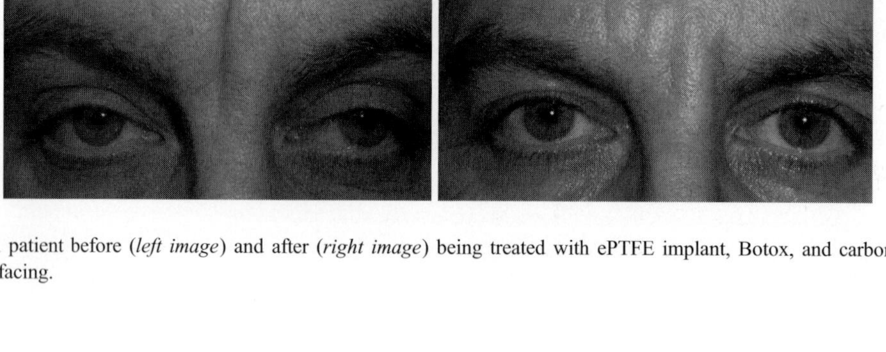

Fig. 21. A patient before (*left image*) and after (*right image*) being treated with ePTFE implant, Botox, and carbon dioxide laser resurfacing.

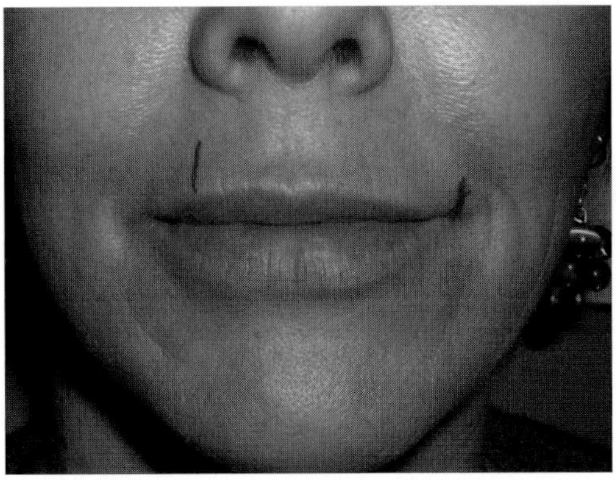

Fig. 22. This case resulted in an implant that was too short. The ends of the implant are marked; it is obvious that the patient's right side is too short.

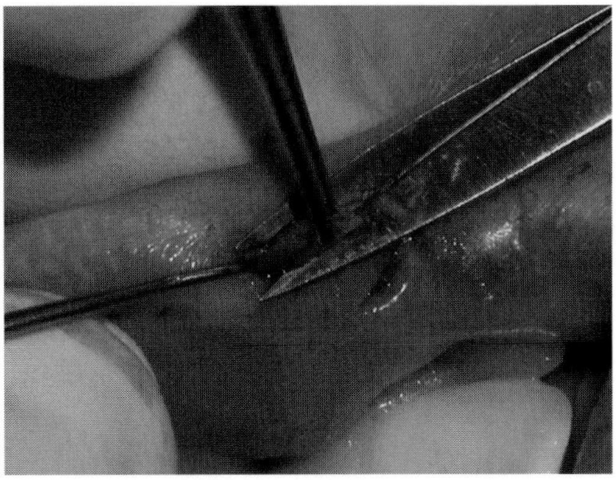

Fig. 24. In the same patient as in Fig. 23, the superficial portion of the implant is trimmed to reduce the palpable and visible bulge.

practitioners frequently treat this area (James Gilmore, MD, personal communication, January 2004). The technique is the same but the implant is obviously smaller.

Complications

As with any procedure, there can exist complications with Advanta implants. I have placed about 50 of these implants and have never seen a complication that involved implant failure, rejection, or infection. Most complications have resulted from improper placement early in the learning curve. I placed implants in the lips that were too short in several patients (Fig. 22). Both of these patients returned for replacement with a longer implant. After placing an upper-lip implant in a flute player, she stated that it affected her ability to play high notes. It was removed and her flute playing returned to normal. One patient experienced prolonged swelling for over a month. Surgical exploration showed the swelling to be a result of a mucous retention phenomenon presumably from injury to the minor salivary glands at the time of placement.

In two patients, the implant tail was placed too superficially (one in the inferior nasolabial fold and one in the lip). The protruding tail was palpable and visible to the patient (Fig. 23). The implant was serviced by making a small incision over the implant tail and retrieving it with a skin hook. The tail was then trimmed and replaced into the incision (Fig. 24). The patients healed without complication and were pleased with the repair.

In cases in which implant removal is necessary, the procedure is easy. An incision is made over one

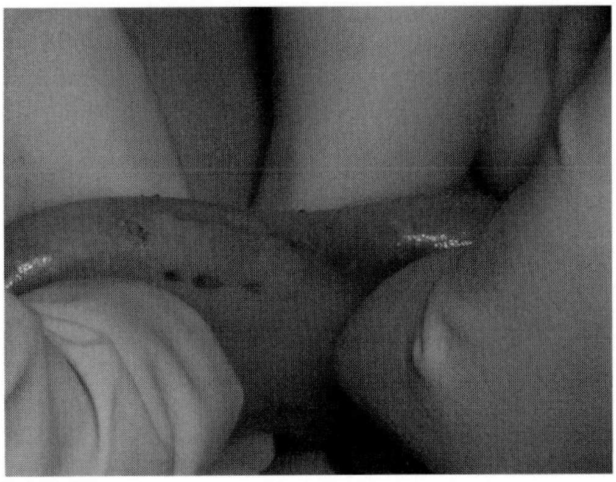

Fig. 23. This implant had the tail placed too superficially in the lip.

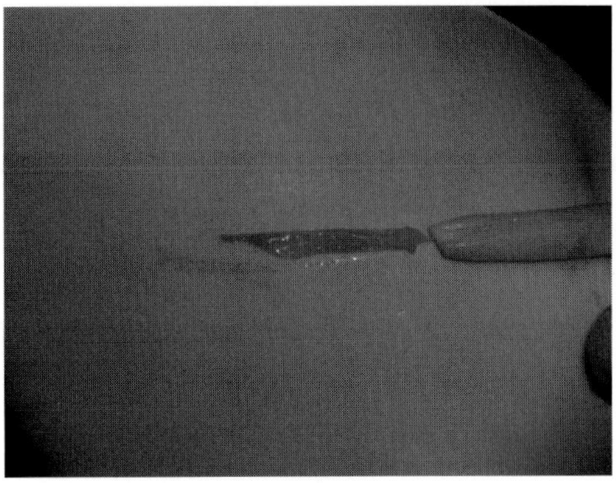

Fig. 25. Advanta implants are easily removed when necessary and may have a thin capsule attached.

of the tails of the implant and the area is bluntly dissected with a hemostat. After the implant tail is visible, it is grasped with a skin hook and then grasped with a hemostat. The lip is firmly grasped and traction is placed on the implant, which will generally extrude. If the implant is adherent, a small freer elevator can be used to dissect along the tunnel to free up the implant. The explant will usually have a small, thin capsule attached (Fig. 25).

Summary

Advanta facial implants represent a new method of ePTFE technology and appear to be different from previous ePTFE products. The implants appear to work well when used for lip augmentation; I have 18 months' experience with this implant. Placement of these implants is simple, and as long as attention is focused on several important factors, the implants are predictable. In my practice, lip augmentation is a frequently requested procedure. Although most of these patients desire injectables such as Restylane, a certain segment of this population desires a more permanent option. Advanta lip implants have proved to be an acceptable option by the surgeon and patient. The complication rate is low and the implants are serviceable. The procedure is reversible without extensive damage to normal tissue. The Advanta facial implant appears to be a useful option in the armamentarium of the cosmetic oral and maxillofacial surgeon.

References

[1] The American Society for Aesthetic Plastic Surgery. Available at: http://www.surgery.org/press/statistics-2003.php. Accessed: May 2004.
[2] Brown LH, Frank PJ. What's new in fillers? J Drugs Dermatol 2003;2(3):250–3.
[3] Niamtu J. Facial implant applications for cosmetic facial surgery. Plastic Surgery Products Novicom Publications 1998;8(5):26–9.
[4] Panossian A, Garner WL. Polytetrafluoroethylene facial implants: 15 years later. Plast Reconstr Surg 2004;113(1):347–9.
[5] Ham J, Miller PJ. Expanded polytetrafluoroethylene implants in rhinoplasty: literature review, operative techniques, and outcome. 6. Facial Plast Surg 2003;19(4):331–9.
[6] Niamtu J. Perioral soft tissue rejuvenation techniques. Compend J 2003;22(11):729–36.
[7] Niamtu J. Alloplastic chin augmentation. Cosmetic facial surgery. Oral Maxillofacial Surg Clin N Am 2000;12(4):765–9.
[8] Niamtu J. Cosmetic surgery options in oral and maxillofacial. J Am Dent Assoc 2000;131(6):756–64.
[9] LaFerriere KA. The adjustable sling in corrective surgery for the aging neck: a promising technique when used with caution. Arch Facial Plast Surg 2003;5(6):502.
[10] Godin M, Costa L, Romo T, et al. Gore-Tex chin implants: a review of 324 cases. Arch Facial Plast Surg 2003;5(3):224–7.
[11] Steinsapir KD. Aesthetic and restorative midface lifting with hand-carved, expanded polytetrafluoroethylene orbital rim implants. Plast Reconstr Surg 2003;111(5):1727–37.
[12] Romo III T, Baskin JZ, Scalfani AP. Augmentation of the cheeks, chin and pre-jowl sulcus, and nasolabial folds. Facial Plast Surg 2001;17(1):67–78.
[13] Choe KS, Stucki-McCormick SU. Chin augmentation. Facial Plast Surg 2000;16(1):45–54.
[14] Constantinides MS, Galli SK, Miller PJ, et al. Malar, submalar, and midfacial implants. Facial Plast Surg 2000;16(1):35–44.
[15] Sclafani AP, Romo III T. Biology and chemistry of facial implants. Facial Plast Surg 2000;16(1):3–6.
[16] Singh S, Baker Jr JL. Use of expanded polytetrafluoroethylene in aesthetic surgery of the face. Clin Plast Surg 2000;27(4):579–93.
[17] Beaty MM. Treatment of neck laxity with a Gore-Tex cervical sling for patients with heavy neck tissues. Facial Plast Surg 2001;17(2):117–22.
[18] Brody HJ. Complications of expanded polytetrafluoroethylene (e-PTFE) facial implant. Dermatol Surg 2001;27(9):792–4.
[19] Maas CS, Denton AB. Synthetic soft tissue substitutes: 2001. Facial Plast Surg Clin N Am 2001;9(2):219–27.
[20] Louis PJ, Cuzalina LA. Alloplastic augmentation of the face. Atlas Oral Maxillofac Surg Clin N Am 2000;8(2):127–91.
[21] Cox III AJ, Wang TD. Skeletal implants in aesthetic facial surgery. Facial Plast Surg 1999;15(1):3–12.
[22] Homsy CA. Complications and toxicities of implantable biomaterials for facial aesthetic and reconstructive surgery. Plast Reconstr Surg 1998;102(5):1766–8.
[23] Lewis RP, Schweitzer J, Odum BC, et al. Sheets, 3-D strands, trimensional (3-D) shapes, and sutures of either reinforced or nonreinforced expanded polytetrafluoroethylene for facial soft-tissue suspension, augmentation, and reconstruction. J Long Term Eff Med Implants 1998;8(1):19–42.
[24] Garner WL. Gore-Tex facial implants. Plastic Surgery Educational Foundation DATA Committee. Plast Reconstr Surg 1997;100(7):1899–900.
[25] Saccoanno F, Bernardi C, Vittorini P. The expanded polytetrafluoroethylene (ePTFE) in the surgical treatment of Parry-Romberg syndrome: case report. Aesthetic Plast Surg 1997;21(5):342–5.
[26] Still II EF. Gore-Tex in facial augmentations. Plast Reconstr Surg 1997;99(5):1468.
[27] Sclafani AP, Thomas JR, Cox AJ, et al. Clinical and histologic response of subcutaneous expanded poly-

tetrafluoroethylene (Gore-Tex) and porous high-density polyethylene (Medpor) implants to acute and early infection. Arch Otolaryngol Head Neck Surg 1997; 123(3):328–36.
[28] Milam SB. Failed implants and multiple operations. Oral Surg Oral Med Oral Pathol Oral Radiol Endod 1997;83(1):156–62.
[29] Maas CS. ePTFE (Gore-Tex) facial augmentation. Plast Reconstr Surg 1996;97(5):1076–7.
[30] Sherris DA, Larrabee Jr WF. Expanded polytetrafluoroethylene augmentation of the lower face. Laryngoscope 1996;106(5 Pt 1):658–63.
[31] Levine B, Berman WE. The current status of expanded polytetrafluoroethylene (Gore-Tex) in facial plastic surgery. Ear Nose Throat J 1995;74(10):681–4.
[32] Schoenrock LD, Chernoff WG. Subcutaneous implantation of Gore-Tex for facial reconstruction. Otolaryngol Clin N Am 1995;28(2):325–40.
[33] Owsley TG, Taylor CO. The use of Gore-Tex for nasal augmentation: a retrospective analysis of 106 patients. Plast Reconstr Surg 1994;94(2):241–8.
[34] Cisneros JL, Singla R. Intradermal augmentation with expanded polytetrafluoroethylene (Gore-Tex) for facial lines and wrinkles. J Dermatol Surg Oncol 1993;19(6): 539–42.
[35] Maas CS, Gnepp DR, Bumpous J. Expanded polytetrafluoroethylene (Gore-Tex soft-tissue patch) in facial augmentation. Arch Otolaryngol Head Neck Surg 1993;119(9):1008–14.
[36] Conrad K, Reifen E. Gore-Tex implant as tissue filler in cheek-lip groove rejuvenation. J Otolaryngol 1992; 21(3):218–22.
[37] Lassus C. Expanded PTFE in the treatment of facial wrinkles. Aesthetic Plast Surg 1991;15(2):167–74.
[38] Neel III HB. Implants of Gore-Tex. Arch Otolaryngol 1983;109(7):427–33.
[39] Hanke CW. A new e-PTFE soft tissue implant for natural-looking augmentation of lips and wrinkles. Dermatol Surg 2002;28:901–8.
[40] Truswell W. A new implant for facial soft tissue augmentation. Arch Facial Plast Surg 2002;4:92–7.
[41] Larrabee WF, Makielski KH. Surgical anatomy of the face. New York: Raven Press; 1993.

ELSEVIER
SAUNDERS

Oral Maxillofacial Surg Clin N Am 17 (2005) 41 – 49

ORAL AND
MAXILLOFACIAL
SURGERY CLINICS
of North America

Botox Injections for Lower Facial Rejuvenation

Michael A.C. Kane, MD*

Department of Plastic Surgery, Manhattan Eye, Ear, and Throat Hospital, New York, NY 10021, USA

Injections of botulinum toxin type A (Botox) are the most frequently performed cosmetic procedure in the United States [1]. Nearly 2.9 million treatments were performed in the United States in 2003. In 15 years, Botox has gone from a relatively obscure specialty drug to being part of our popular culture. It is now a verb in the dictionary, a subject for numerous sitcoms, part of our everyday vocabulary, and even an issue in presidential elections. Despite its popularity, the drug is still widely misunderstood, especially in regard to its use in the lower face. When injected properly in selected patients, Botox is an excellent rejuvenative tool in the perioral area.

Botox is a fully sequenced 1295 amino acid chain metalloprotease. It consists of a 97-kd heavy chain connected by a disulfide bond to a 52-kd light chain. The heavy chain binds to the cell membrane of the distal axon, which allows the light chain to penetrate the cell membrane into the cytoplasm. After it is inside the cell, it cleaves synaptosomal-associated protein 25, an essential protein in the mechanism that allows the acetylcholine-containing vesicles to fuse with the cell membrane, thus depositing the neurotransmitter into the synapse. By blocking this pathway, Botox prevents the presynaptic release of acetylcholine to the corresponding motor endplates. Although it is often said that Botox does nothing directly to the skin and acts only on the muscles beneath it, this is clearly not true. Clearly, Botox only directly affects the nerve. Depending on the dose injected, Botox can produce a full range of effects, from mild weakness to full paralysis of a given muscle. At times, Botox is even used on selective parts of a single muscle. This exacting control is necessary to achieve facial rejuvenation while minimizing complications in the lower face. Clinically, the rejuvenating effects of Botox persist for approximately 3 months in the lower face after initial injection, but the duration of action typically increases after multiple treatments [2].

The first study to describe the therapeautic application of the toxin (in rhesus monkeys) was published by Dr. Alan Scott (an ophthalmologist) and colleagues [3] in 1973. Scott's [4] first publication that described its use in humans for strabismus appeared in 1980. The first study detailing the use of Botox for cosmetic reasons was published in 1992 [5]. Soon thereafter, other uses in the upper face and neck were described in the medical literature [6–12]. To this day, these are established and widely accepted areas for Botox injection. The use of Botox in the perioral area is still considered controversial at best and something to be altogether avoided at worst on the Botox/facial rejuvenation lecture circuit. Instead, the use of fillers in the lower face and the use of Botox for the upper face are stressed. I believe that this separation of treatments is arbitrary and often not in the patient's best interest but more in the comfort zone of the patient's physician. In selected patients, Botox is an excellent treatment for nasal labial folds, perioral rhytids, marionette's lines, dimpled chins, and downturned oral commissures.

The pathogenesis of the wrinkle is important in determining how effective Botox will be in effacing it

* 630 Park Avenue, New York, NY 10021.
E-mail address: michaelkanemd@earthlink.net

doi:10.1016/j.coms.2004.09.003

[13]. When the wrinkle is primarily caused by severe changes in the skin caused by sun damage [14], smoking [15], and dermal thinning, the effectiveness of Botox may be limited. When the rhytid is primarily caused by overhanging ptotic skin, surgery will probably be the most effective treatment. When the rhytid is primarily or at least significantly caused by muscular action deforming the overlying skin, Botox can be an extremely effective treatment in the lower face.

Nasolabial folds

I first began using Botox for cosmetic reasons in 1991. I attended the 25th meeting of the American Society for Aesthetic Plastic Surgery in Los Angeles in May 1992 at which Joel Pessa [16] from the University of Texas presented a paper detailing the different effects of the mimetic muscles on facial movements and rhytids. Fresh cadaver heads were used and, after raising the skin, a dynamometer was attached to the different mimetic muscles to determine their effects on facial expression. As expected, the muscle most responsible for the smile was the zygomaticus major. The muscle least important for the smile was the levator labii superioris alequae nasii. The levator labii superioris alequae nasii muscle, however, was the muscle most responsible for formation of the medial nasolabial fold. The presenter then said that he was beginning to surgically divide this muscle in selected patients [17]. Sitting in the audience, this made sense, but I was fearful of permanently weakening this muscle. If a patient were to be unhappy with the treatment, then there would be no effective recourse. I thought that this muscle would be an excellent one to inject with Botox to soften the medial nasolabial folds. If the patient were to be unhappy with the result, then the treatment would only be temporary and would return to preinjection status within a few months. If satisfied, the patient could continue to have this muscle injected regularly along with other areas of the face.

In May 1992, I began injecting this muscle in patients. Of the first 25 patients injected, 16 returned for repeat injection. Although this treatment yielded a satisfaction rate of 64%, I was concerned about the other 36%. All of these patients were unhappy with their smile after injection. Although the levator labii superioris alequae nasii muscle has a minimal contribution to the smile, its contribution is not nonexistent. This muscle is responsible for the final 3 to 4 mm of central upper-lip elevation [18]. The dissatisfied patients were almost uniformly unhappy with the loss of elevation of the central upper lip.

Rubin [19] published an article detailing different smile patterns in 1974. This classic article described how the smile mechanism works, which mimetic muscles dominate, and how these muscles act in concert to form discrete patterns. Different smiling patterns also have been described for crow's feet [20]. The most common smile pattern, which Rubin [19] termed the Mona Lisa smile, is present in 63% of the population. When smiling, the patient raises the commissures to the highest point of the smile, and the dominant muscle in these patients is the zygomaticus major. The next most common pattern is the canine smile pattern. Its dominant muscle is the levator labii superioris, and the smile is characterized by raising the central upper lip higher than the commissures. The canine smile pattern is present in 35% of the population. The least common pattern is the full denture smile, which is characterized by simultaneous firing of the upper-lip elevators and lower-lip depressors. Of these initial 25 patients, those who were unhappy with their postinjection smiles were strong Mona Lisa–smile patients. Post injection, they were left with exaggerated Mona Lisa smiles, with the commissures significantly higher than the central upper lip. These patients could not afford to lose any central upper-lip elevation.

By contrast, the happiest patients were strong canine-smile patients. They had exaggerated elevation of the central upper lip before injection and were glad to be converted to Mona Lisa smile patterns after injection. All patients had softening of their medial nasolabial folds.

An exaggerated version of the canine-smile patient is the patient with the gummy smile (Fig. 1). There are many descriptions of surgical procedures in the literature to address this problem [21,22]. These patients frequently do not smile for photographs and cover their mouth with their hands while laughing. They also tend to have sharp and often asymmetric medial nasolabial folds. These patients benefit most from injection of the levator labii superioris alequae nasii. Their upper lip is lowered to cover their gingiva, and their sharp medial nasal labial folds are softened.

The levator labii superioris alequae nasii is the most medial of the mimetic muscles. It is found in the groove between the nasal bone and maxilla. There is a wide dose range (from a total of 3.75 to 15 U Botox) for injection of this muscle. Most patients fall in the 5- to 7.5-U range total for both sides. Patients with severely gummy smiles are nearly always asymmetric, and one side should be injected at a higher dose than the other. Patients must be informed

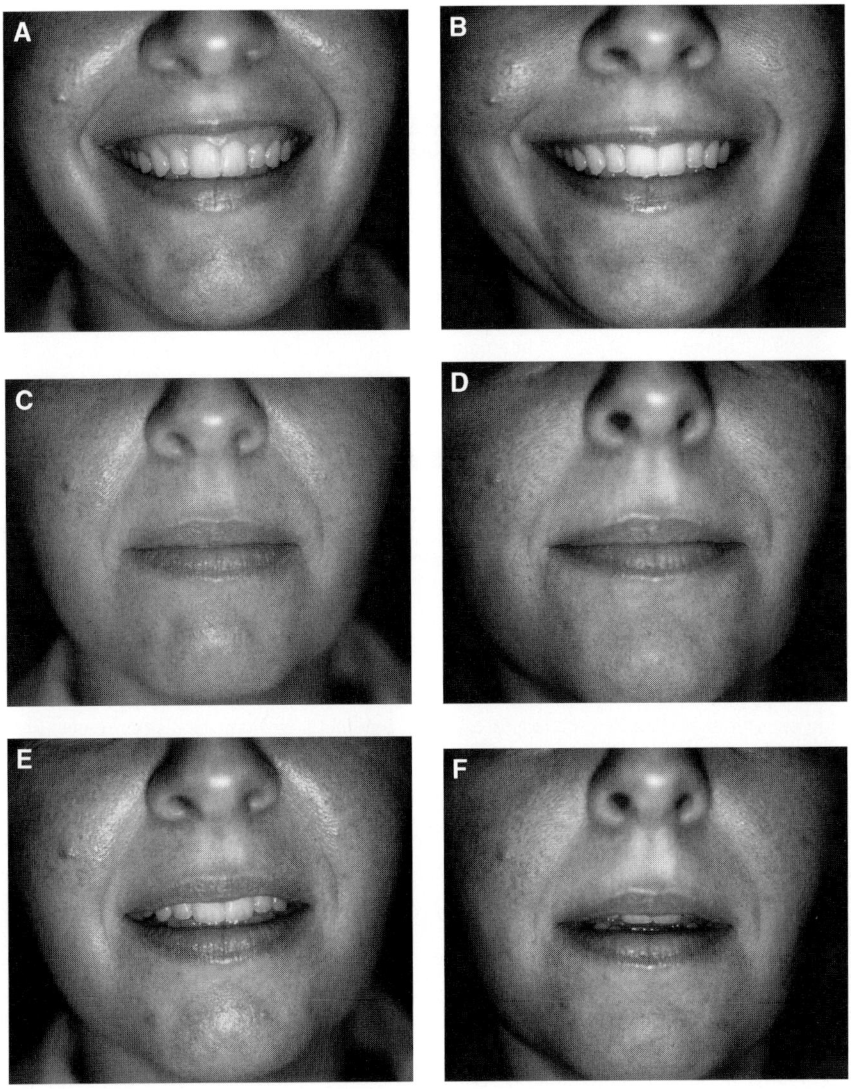

Fig. 1. The patient is a 34-year-old woman who complained of a gummy smile for many years. (*A*) Preinjection, she had a mildly asymmetric gummy smile (most gummy smiles are more asymmetric than this) with sharp medial nasolabial folds (left slightly higher than right). She had symmetric Botox injection of 7.5 U total to her levator labii superioris alequae nasi muscles. (*B*) Her postinjection smiling photograph reveals a lowering of her upper lip centrally more than laterally. The height of her central upper lip now has a better relationship to the height of her commissures. She is nearly in the Mona Lisa smile category (still slightly canine). Her medial nasolabial folds also are greatly improved. In fact, her lower nasolabial folds, or parentheses lines, are slightly exaggerated. These patients sometimes receive concomitant filler injection to the parentheses lines. The patient (*C*) before and (*D*) after injection, in repose, with the mouth closed. Even without smiling, there is an obvious improvement in the medial nasolabial fold. The lightly etched line on the patient's left is removed above the parentheses line, which attests to the strong pull even at rest of the levator labii superioris alequae nasi in the patient with a gummy smile. Such an improvement at rest is not usually seen in the standard canine smile patient. The patient (*E*) before and (*F*) after injections in repose in natural posture. When focused on the perioral area, it may appear as though the patient is smiling; however, she is not. This position was her natural resting position, which she found unattractive. The resting tone of her levator labii superioris nasi muscles has been reduced, allowing her upper lip to rest in a lower, although still not closed, position.

of the coming change to their smile pattern (lowering of the central upper lip) before injection.

Perioral lines

Radial, perioral wrinkles form around the mouth for a variety of reasons. Environmental factors, ultraviolet radiation, smoking, and thinning of the skin with aging contribute to the intrinsic aging of the perioral skin. Sphincteric action of the orbicularis oris deforms the densely adherent overlying skin thousands of times per day, creating the basis for the radial lines that appear more readily in older, thin skin. In addition, lips lose volume during the aging process. Thus, there is less "stuffing" in the lips, which also contributes to deeper rhytids. To maximize perioral rejuvenation with no downtime to the patient, all three causes must be addressed.

Sun avoidance, cessation of smoking, protection with sunscreens, and application of topical products such as alpha hydroxy acids, vitamin C, and retinoids can be used to address the intrinsic aging of the skin. Filler materials such as bovine collagen, human collagen, and hyaluronic acids can be used to address the loss of volume of the lips. When the underlying deforming force of the orbicularis oris is not addressed, however, rejuvenation will be suboptimal.

In my practice, skin care is stressed to every cosmetic patient. The most common office procedure performed for rejuvenation of the perioral rhytids is Restylane injection. Injection of Restylane restores volume to the lips and can be used to address individual deeper rhytids. Although Restylane can achieve an excellent improvement on its own, if the underlying deforming force of the orbicularis oris (the root cause of the rhytids) is not addressed, then the result will not be as good and will not last as long. There are three groups of patients in my practice who benefit from orbicularis oris injection with Botox. The first group of candidates for injection consists of patients who are happy with the effects of Botox in other areas of the face who ask whether Botox can be used to make their perioral rhytids better. The risks, benefits, and alternatives are discussed before these patients are injected. The second group of patients includes those who desire perioral rejuvenation but absolutely refuse to have their lips made any larger. This request is common in New York but perhaps less so in southern California and Florida. The third and largest group is made up of patients who desire the maximal improvement in their perioral appearance without the downtime associated with chemical peels, dermabrasion, laser resurfacing, or surgery. These patients are instructed on proper skin care, have appropriate injection of filler material, and have relaxation of the sphincter with injection of Botox. Injection with filler material alone is limiting. In the older patient with severe radial rhytids, a great deal of filler material would be required to maximally improve these lines (Fig. 2). The amount of filler material required would make the patient look quite strange. In my practice, I inject a judicious amount of filler material to restore volume and fill radial lines but not so much as to make the patient look "done" or to have strangely large lips. Then, the sphincter is gently weakened with an even application of Botox.

My current dose range per lip of Botox is 2 to 7 U. Most patients fall in the category of 2 to 4 U per lip. The philtrum is rarely injected because it rarely develops sharp radial lines due to the unique skin in this area. The remainder of the upper lip is injected diffusely with dilute toxin using a threading technique 2 to 3 mm above the vermilion border. My standard dilution is 4 mL of nonpreserved normal saline per 100-U vial. When injecting a lip, the proper dose is drawn into the syringe; however, this small volume is difficult to distribute evenly throughout a lip. Therefore, additional normal saline is drawn into the syringe so that an appropriate volume is present that can then be evenly injected throughout the sphincter. If the upper and lower lips are to be treated, then they should be retreated at the same time. Dosages are based on apparent muscle mass and not the depth of the rhytids in the skin. Beware the elderly female patient with severe radial rhytids but decreased muscle mass in her lip. Four to 5 U of Botox in this patient's lip would probably lead to speech problems and, potentially, oral incompetence. These patients must be warned in advance that they will feel a bit weak or strange after injection. Usually, this sensation is gone in my patients within 2 weeks.

I have developed this threading technique over many years and through careful analysis of photographs of prior patients. When examining before and after pictures in repose, the area of least improvement usually is the area of maximal motion when patients are instructed to purse their lips. It is my goal during injection to effect a diffuse yet perfectly even relaxation of the sphincter, which is very difficult to do when placing several serial puncture injections around the sphincter. Despite some diffusion of the toxin in the direction of the orbicularis oris muscle fibers, there often are areas of relative weakness versus relative strength juxtaposed around the sphincter when a serial puncture method is used. This situation can result in a strange appearance while

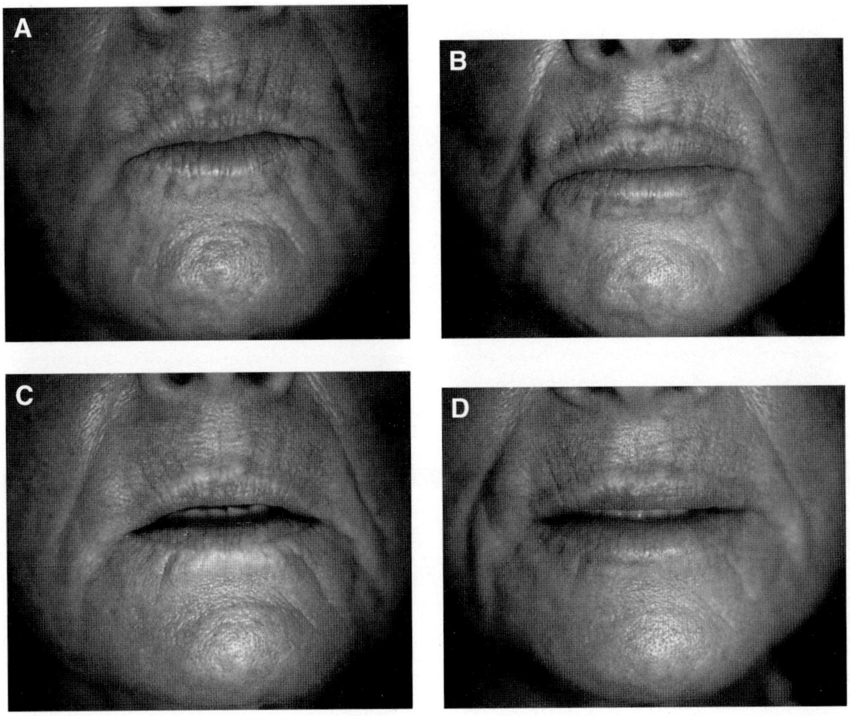

Fig. 2. The patient is a 71-year-old woman who complained of deep perioral rhytids that were minimally responsive to prior single-modality treatments. She is shown pursing her lips (*A*) before and (*B*) after Botox injection of 3.5 U to her upper lip, 2 U to her lower lip, and 2 U to each depressor anguli oris muscle. She also had a total of 2 mL zyplast bovine collagen to her lips only. The radiating rhytids around her mouth were not injected. Note that she can no longer strongly purse her lips but does not have a problem with oral competence. The author injected her first with the collagen, using as much material as possible before making the lips overly large. Note how the left upper lip is more evenly weakened than the right. A subtle upturn of her commissures also is seen. The same patient in repose (*C*) before and (*D*) after injection. The lips are full but not overdone. Note the eversion of the lower lip. The area of least improvement (right upper lip) corresponds to the area with more motion, as seen in the animated photos. Strong upturn of the commissures is noted in repose due to her depressor anguli oris injection. Note the improvement of the lower-lip rhytids and marionette's lines without filler material in these areas.

pursing the lips and often will result in less than optimal rejuvenation.

Mentalis

In the selected patient, injection of the mentalis muscle can rejuvenate the chin area [23]; however, it is one of the trickiest muscles to inject because overinjection of the mentalis will surely lead to oral incompetence. When saying certain sounds or when closing their mouth in repose, many patients dimple the skin overlying their mentalis muscle. These patients are ideal for rejuvenation by injection of this muscle. Another group of patients who have had one or more (frequently multiple) chin implant procedures often have some disinsertion of the mentalis, with compensatory hypertrophy and dimpling of the overlying skin. These patients also benefit from Botox injection with or without accompanying mentalis resuspension.

The mentalis muscle is attached to its overlying skin with thick fibrous septae. These septae transmit the topography of the mentalis muscle to the skin above. Therefore, when injecting this muscle, I try to inject only the superficial mentalis, leaving the deep mentalis fully functional. By smoothing the superficial mentalis, the overlying skin also is smoothed, which allows the deep mentalis to function fully and protect oral competence. Clearly, the dominant risk during mentalis injection is overinjection of the mentalis muscle, which could lead to full lower-incisor show and to oral incompetence. Care should

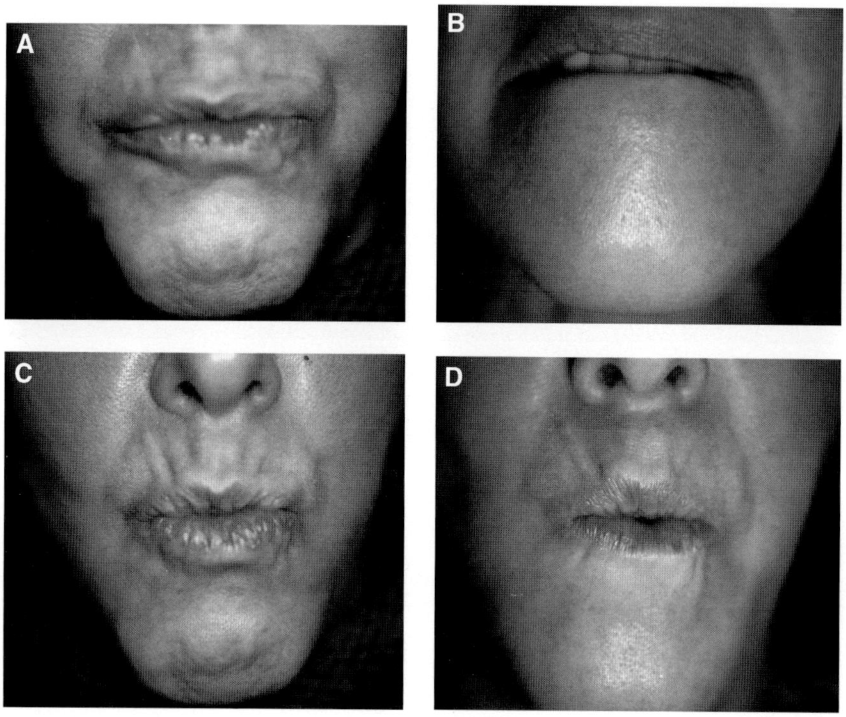

Fig. 3. This patient requested rejuvenation of the lower face. She did not like the dimples on her chin that would appear during speech and mouth closure. (*A*) Before injection, she had obvious dimpling over the mentum when raising her lower lip. She had 5 U of Botox injected into her superficial mentalis. Care was taken not to inject the deep portion of the muscle. (*B*) After injection, despite straining maximally, she cannot reproduce the dimpling. The change in her orbicularis oris and depressor anguli oris action also is obvious. The patient is seen pursing her lips (*C*) before and (*D*) after 2 U of Botox were injected into each lip. Note the general easing of rhytids. The rhytids of the left upper lip are improved more (due to less motion) than the rhytids of the right upper lip. The lower lip is more evenly improved, which illustrates how difficult it is to evenly inject the entirety of the sphincter (except for the philtrum). The patient is shown (*E*) before and (*F*) after injection of 7.5 U of Botox into her depressor anguli oris muscles in four evenly divided doses. The first injection on each side is where the diagonally aligned rhytid (parallel to the border of the mandible) appears while retracting the lower lip. The second injection is placed midway between this point and the border of the mandible. The injection points are indicated in Fig. 3E by the arrows on the patient's right. Note the smoothness of this area and the inability to create these wrinkles post injection. The patient is shown in repose (natural posture) (*G*) before and (*H*) after the previous injections. The level of the upper lip remains the same but the lower lip rides higher, eliminating lower-incisor show. The commissures are upturned. The upper lip appears more full (no fillers were used). (*I*) Before and (*J*) after the previous injections, the patient still has a pleasing smile. The lower lip is mildly elevated and the upper lip appears more full after mild sphincter weakening. The patient is shown in repose with the mouth closed (*K*) before and (*L*) after the injections. The most obvious change is in the mentum, which not only is less dimpled but also less boxy in appearance. Patients with hypertrophic mentalis muscles often have a square, boxy appearance due to the width and size of this muscle. This muscle can be shaped with Botox. The commissures are up, and the early hollows beneath them are improved. The lips appear more full, and the proportions of the area are more aesthetic.

especially be taken in patients with extremely dimpled skin over the mentalis. This dimpling is not a random event in most patients. The skin of these patients is so dimpled because they often have a hypertrophic mentalis muscle, as strong function of this muscle is necessary to maintain oral competence. Therefore, the patients most likely to be helped by mentalis injection are also those predisposed to develop a complication from it.

My current dosage range of Botox for the entire mentalis is 2.5 to 12.5 U. Most patients require close to 5 U in their superficial mentalis to smooth this area. Immediately before injection, patients are asked to push their lower lip upward against their upper lip

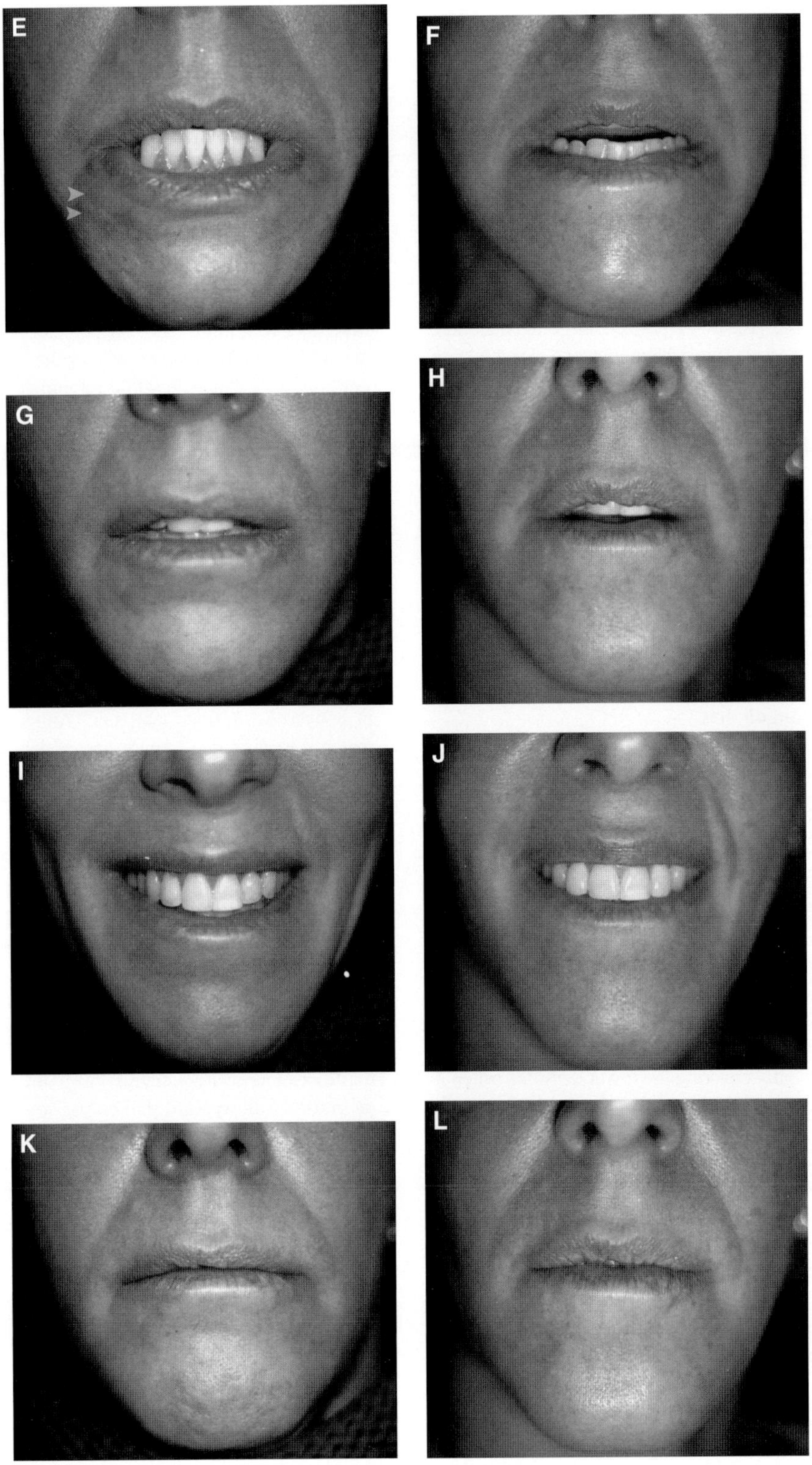

Fig. 3 (*continued*).

as strongly as possible. This action strains the mentalis muscle, and areas of contour irregularity can be seen and, thus, injected. The injection is aimed parallel to the skin surface along the superficial aspect of the muscle. Although impossible to carry out (or check), I aim for the superficial muscle/muscle fascia plane while injecting here. This technique is the one I also use when injecting a disinserted mentalis after chin augmentation surgery [24]. Approximately 30% of patients will need a small touch up injection after their initial injection. I prefer this process to the risk of giving too large an injection, which could result in oral incompetence. The real risk of drooling outweighs the theoretic risk of increasing the possibility of resistance to the drug. Frequently, I will inject the depressor anguli oris at the same time I inject the mentalis muscle. If the lower-lip elevator is overly weakened, then the lower lip sometimes sits at a lower level in repose, revealing the lower teeth and gingiva and changing the smile. To prevent this situation, I frequently inject the lower-lip depressors while injecting the mentalis to balance lower-lip position (Fig. 3).

Depressor anguli oris

Of all the muscles suitable for Botox injection in lower face, the depressor anguli oris is the one in my practice with the lowest risk and nearly universal acceptance among patients. This muscle and its dermal insertions help to form the marionettes lines that are so troubling to patients. This muscle also assists gravity and in pulling down the oral commissures, a sign of aging that is troubling to most patients. In the rare times that I believe I have over-injected this muscle, oral incompetence is not a side effect. Rather, the lower lip rides in an elevated position, frequently covering the lower dentition when it had been exposed during repose before injection. In fact, if the lower orbicularis oris or mentalis has been overly weakened and oral competence challenged, injecting the depressor anguli oris can alleviate this side effect in patients. This muscle also is the muscle to inject on the contralateral side of a marginal mandibular nerve injury to regain facial symmetry [25].

The depressor anguli oris is a triangularly shaped muscle, with its base along the caudal border of the mandible and its apex inserting into the modiolus. The key to safely injecting this muscle, in my experience, has been to avoid trying to inject its apex. At the cephalad portion of the muscle, there are few muscle fibers remaining. Most likely, attempted cephalad injection of this muscle will result in bolus injection of the lateral orbicularis oris of the lower lip, which clearly can lead to oral incompetence. I inject the mid portion and base of the muscle instead. With the dentition occluded, patients are asked to show me their lower teeth. This nearly always elicits a small rhytid below the commissure parallel to the caudal border of the mandible. Each muscle is injected in two sites. The first injection lies at the dermal insertion at the mid portion of the depressor anguli oris. The second injection point is midway between the first injection point and the caudal border of the mandible and effectively weakens the mid and lower portions of the muscle while minimizing the chance of diffusion of the toxin into the orbicularis oris of the lower lip.

If the marionette's lines are caused by a large amount of hanging, ptotic skin or a large discrepancy between the amount of subcutaneous fat lateral to the line and that over the mentum, then minimal improvement will be seen. Large amounts of ptotic skin should be addressed with surgery. Smaller amounts can be camouflaged with filler materials. Filler materials also can be used to camouflage a subcutaneous fat discrepancy. Botox is commonly used in concert with filler materials. Although the filler material ameliorates a sharp line of demarcation, the Botox minimizes the downward pull on the dermal insertions of the muscle, raises the oral commissures, and increases the duration of action of the filler material. The cosmetic benefits of weakening this muscle are readily apparent when one considers the appearance of a patient after a mental nerve block. Due to its proximity, in my hands, the depressor anguli oris invariably becomes paralyzed after mental nerve injection. Even allowing for the beneficial effect of swelling and added volume, when the patient is upright, there is a dramatic improvement in the lower face. The patient's lower lip rides up and the muscle's downward pull on the commissures and marionette's lines is gone. One of the most difficult problems in facial aesthetic surgery is the severely etched lines that form below the commissures. Even with a well-done face-lift, laser resurfacing, and filler materials, these rhytids can remain quite prominent. Treating the depressor anguli oris over a period of years can prevent these deep lines from forming.

Summary

Botox is an excellent adjunct for rejuvenation of the lower face. It should be considered in addition to surgery, resurfacing, skin care, and filler materials to improve the appearance of the lower face. Excellent control and familiarity with the toxin is essential before injecting these rewarding although technically more demanding areas of the face. In the perioral area, a few stray units in the wrong muscle or wrong portion of a muscle will guarantee an unhappy patient; this is not an area for the novice injector. When first beginning to inject the lower face, lower doses and more frequent touch-ups are better than larger initial doses and severe complications.

References

[1] American Society of Aesthetic Plastic Surgeons. 2003 national plastic surgery statistics: cosmetic and reconstructive patients. Available at: http://www.plasticsurgery.org/public_education/2003statistics.cfm. Accessed: July 13, 2004.

[2] Kane MAC. Atrophy after repeated botox injections. Paper presented at the American Society for Aesthetic Plastic Surgery Meeting. Los Angeles (CA), May 2, 1998.

[3] Scott AB, Rosenbaum A, Collins CC. Pharmacologic weakening of extraocular muscles. Invest Ophthalmol Vis Sci 1973;12:924–7.

[4] Scott AB. Botulinum toxin injection into extraocular muscles as an alternative to strabismus surgery. Ophthalmology 1980;87:1044.

[5] Carruthers JDA, Carruthers JA. Treatment of glabellar frown lines with *Clostridium botulinum* A exotoxin. Dermatol Surg 1992;18:17–21.

[6] Blitzer A, Brin MF, Keen MS, et al. Botulinum toxin for the treatment of hyperfunctional lines of the face. Arch Otolaryngol Head Neck Surg 1993;119:1018.

[7] Keen M, Blitzer A, Aviv J, et al. Botulinum toxin A for hyperkinetic facial lines: results of double blind, placebo controlled study. Plast Reconstr Surg 1994; 94:94.

[8] Ascher B, Klap P, Marion MH, et al. Botulinum toxin in the treatment of frontoglabellar and periorbital wrinkles. Ann Chir Plast Esthet 1995;40:67.

[9] Garcia A, Fulton Jr JE. Cosmetic denervation of the muscles of facial expression with botulinum toxin: a dose response study. Dermatol Surg 1996;22:39.

[10] Carruthers A, Kiene K, Carruthers J. Botulinum A exotoxin use in clinical dermatology. J Am Acad Dermatol 1996;34:788.

[11] Lowe NJ, Wirder JM. Botulinum toxin for hyperkinetic facial lines: a placebo controlled study. Cosm Dermatol 1998;8:16.

[12] Kane MAC. Nonsurgical treatment of platysmal bands with injection of botulinum toxin A. Plast Reconst Surg 1999;103:656.

[13] Kligman AM, Zheng P, Lavker RM. The anatomy and pathogenesis of wrinkles. Br J Dermatol 1985; 113(1):37.

[14] Bhawan J, Andersen W, Lee J, et al. Photoaging versus intrinsic aging: a morphologic assessment of facial skin. J Cutan Pathol 1995;22(2):154.

[15] Daniell HW. Smoker's wrinkles: a study in the epidemiology of "crow's feet. Ann Intern Med 1971; 75:873.

[16] Pessa J. Independent effect of various facial mimetic muscles on the nasolabial fold. Presented at the 25th meeting of the American Society for Aesthetic Plastic Surgery. Los Angeles (CA), May 1992.

[17] Pessa J. Improving the acute nasolabial angle and medial nasolabial fold by levator alae muscle resection. Ann Plast Surg 1992;29:23.

[18] Kane MAC. The effect of botulinum toxin injections on the nasolabial fold. Plast Reconst Surg 2003; 112:66s.

[19] Rubin LR. The anatomy of a smile: its importance in the treatment of facial paralysis. Plast Reconst Surg 1974;53:384.

[20] Kane MAC. Classification of crow's feet patterns among caucasian women: the key to individualizing treatment. Plast Reconst Surg 2003;112:33s.

[21] Litton C, Fournier P. Simple correction of the gummy smile. Plast Reconst Surg 1979;63:372.

[22] Ellenbogen R, Swara N. The improvement of the gummy smile using the implant spacer technique. Plast Reconst Surg 1984;12:16.

[23] Kane MAC. A new use for botox—the labiomental area. Paper presented at the 33rd annual meeting of the American Society for Aesthetic Plastic Surgery. Orlando (FL), May 13, 2000.

[24] Zide B. Chin surgery. III: revelations. Plast Reconst Surg 2003;111:1542.

[25] Kane MAC. Botox for the treatment of sugical compliations. Paper presented at the University of Toronto Plastic Surgery Symposium. Toronto, Ontario, April 4, 2002.

ELSEVIER
SAUNDERS

Oral Maxillofacial Surg Clin N Am 17 (2005) 51 – 63

ORAL AND
MAXILLOFACIAL
SURGERY CLINICS
of North America

Minimally Invasive Percutaneous Collagen Induction

Desmond Fernandes, MB, BCh, FRCS(Edin)

The Shirnel Clinic and Department of Plastic Reconstructive Surgery, University of Cape Town, 822 Fountain Medical Centre, Heerengracht, Cape Town 8001, South Africa

We live in a time when more people are living to a greater age than ever before. At the same time, there is an accent on youth such that our patients are asking us to make them look as young as possible. Obviously, surgery helps restructure the face into a more youthful shape, but the old skin remains. Today, many patients come before they need surgery, searching for a rapid solution that will make them look 10 years younger. How do we help our older cosmetic patients or the much younger men and women who want to prolong their tenure in a youthful bracket?

This quest for younger-looking skin has spawned many different topical techniques that share the same principle of damaging the skin to cause fibrosis. The fibrosis then causes tightening of the skin. Historically, skin peels were the first method of skin rejuvenation. The principle of peeling is to destroy the epidermis partially or almost completely to damage the fibroblasts and dermal structures. This damage then sets up an inflammatory response proportional to the damage, which results in the deposition of collagen. Peeling sacrifices the epidermis to achieve the desired result. The experience with partial-depth burns misled many into believing that the epidermis is a self-renewing organ that rapidly grows over the damaged area, which is why peels became progressively more destructive for the epidermis (eg, the deep phenol peel) until the accumulated problems forced clinicians to recognize that smoother skin comes at a very heavy price for many patients and also leads to a significant thinning of the skin many years later. The proponents of peeling looked only at the increase of collagen in the papillary and reticular dermis but did not pay any attention to the epidermis. The epidermis suffered by becoming less undulating due to the destruction of the dermal papillae and subsequent impaired nourishment and, in turn resulted in a thinner epidermis with fewer cells in the stratum spinosum than before treatment. The stratum corneum is then less likely to act as an efficient barrier, so it is not surprising that many patients feel that their skin is too dry for years after the treatment. Consequently, hydration of the dermis also is affected.

Lighter peels (eg, Jessner's and trichloracetic acid (TCA)) were introduced, but the tightening of skin was less effective. For some reason, which is difficult to understand, clinicians in the late 1980s turned to laser to destroy the epidermis even more thoroughly to tighten the skin. We were told that laser would not present the same problems as the heavy phenol peels and that skin color and texture would be superior. Smoothing skin is still most effectively done by CO_2 laser through the aggressive heat damage that is caused. No other technique can match it, but at the same time, CO_2 laser causes the most complications. A significant problem is that deep treatments like this stimulate fibrosis rather than new, naturally oriented collagen formation. This fibrosis may result in a much whiter reflectance from the dermis, giving the skin an unnatural pallor. The sad fact is that several years after the treatment, the collagen will be

The author, a plastic and reconstructive surgeon practicing in Cape Town, is the medical consultant for Environ Cosmeceutics International and Vivida Closed Corporation (c.c.), Cape Town, South Africa. Vivida c.c. is the manufacturer of the Environ Roll-Cit. Dr. Fernandes has a financial interest in both of these companies.

E-mail address: des@environ.co.za

1042-3699/05/$ – see front matter
doi:10.1016/j.coms.2004.09.004

resorbed—as all scar collagen is—and fine wrinkles will start to show as a result of the thin epidermis with no dermal papillae. The impaired hydration of the skin means that it is not as plump as it could be and can look atrophic due to this excessive destruction.

Why destroy the epidermis to make the skin smoother? The epidermis is an extremely complex, highly specialized organ. It may be only 0.2 mm thick but it is our sole protection from the environment. We should never damage the epidermis unless the risk of leaving the epidermis intact is greater than the risk of removing it. Wrinkles are hardly a good excuse to destroy this wonderfully complex interface that we have with the world. Whatever we do, we should try to ensure that the basic normal architecture of the skin is never altered. To rejuvenate facial skin and really look young, we need a perfect epidermis with natural dermal papillae, good hydration, normal color, and normal resilience.

The problem with most treatments that are used is that only the face can successfully be treated. In addition, if the result after one treatment is inadequate, then a repeated treatment cannot easily be done. Clinicians have concentrated on rejuvenating the face, with the result that we get patients with a younger-looking face but with older hands, arms, and trunk. We need to treat not only the face but the hands, arms, trunk, and legs. Laser, however, has extremely limited indications for areas other than the face. Laser treatment is not real rejuvenation and will not satisfy patients who are looking for a more complete rejuvenation.

This article is devoted to a technique that lends itself to treatment of the face and the body to achieve collagen induction. Although this technique may seem new, we have had centuries of experience with the technique of tattooing, but in this case, there is no pigment used. There are now a growing number of clinicians who believe that we can get closer to our patients' dreams of rejuvenation by pricking skin with needles to get percutaneous collagen induction (PCI).

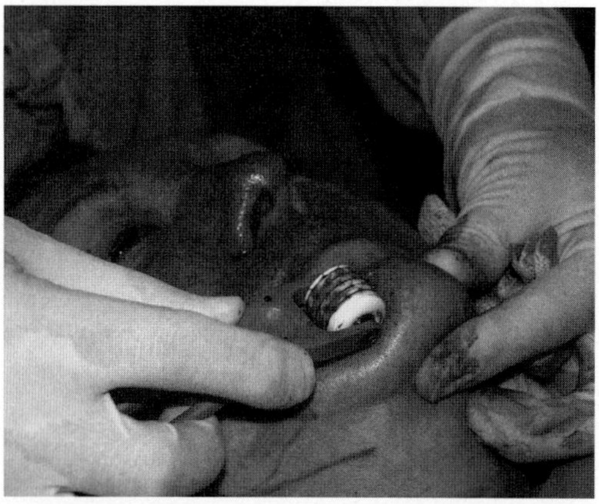

Fig. 1. Needling the face for refining wrinkles using the special tool designed for PCI.

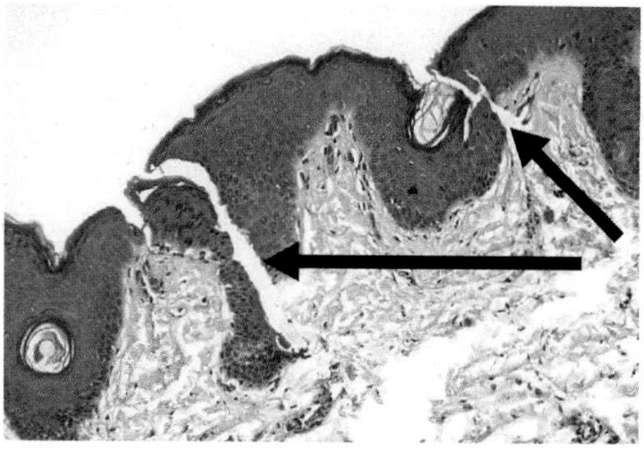

Fig. 2. Histologic section of skin showing puncture sites where the needle has penetrated (*arrows*) and generally divided cells from each other rather than cutting through the cells. The tracts are curved, reflecting the path of the needle as it rolls into and then out of the skin. The holes are about four cells wide and will heal rapidly. Note that the epidermis and particularly the stratum corneum is intact except for these tiny holes (hematoxylin-eosin, original magnification × 40).

Principles of the needling technique

Orentreich and Orentreich [1] described "subcision" as a way of building up connective tissue beneath retracted scars and wrinkles. The author [2], simultaneously and independently, used a similar technique to treat the upper lip by sticking a 15-gauge needle into the skin and then tunneling under the wrinkles in various directions, parallel to the skin surface. The lip wrinkles were improved in many cases, but the problem was that bleeding caused severe and unacceptable bruising, which sometimes resulted in hard nodules. Camirand and Doucet [3] treated scars with a tattoo gun to "needle abrade" them. Although this technique can be used on extensive areas, it is laboriously slow and the holes in the epidermis are too close and too shallow. These techniques work because the needles break old collagen strands in the most superficial layer of the dermis that tether scars or wrinkles. It is presumed that this process promotes removal of damaged collagen and induces more collagen immediately under the epidermis. The author believes that the standard technique of tattooing is too superficial to give good effects for thicker scars or for stimulating collage-

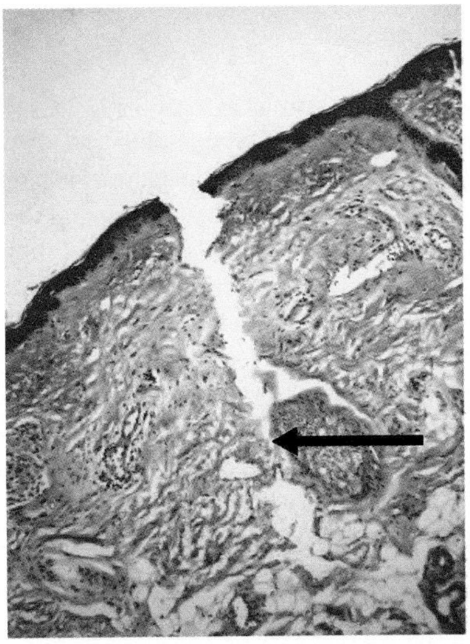

Fig. 3. Histologic section shows that the needle tract penetrates to a depth of about 1.5 to 2 mm through the papillary dermis into the reticular dermis (hematoxylin-eosin, original magnification × 40).

nosis in the reticular dermis. Needles need to penetrate relatively deeply to stimulate the production of elastin fibers oriented from the deep layers of the dermis to the surface. Based on these principles, the author designed a special tool for PCI [4] (Fig. 1).

Indications for needling

Indications for percutaneous collagen induction

1. To restore skin tightness in the early stages of facial aging. This procedure is relatively minor and can safely be recommended. Some patients who are worried about cosmetic surgery may be satisfied with simple PCI. The neck, arms, abdomen, thighs, and areas between the breasts and buttocks also can be treated. Upper-lip creases can respond very well to needling (Figs. 2–4) but may give an even better result when combined with fat grafts.
2. Fine wrinkles are an excellent indication for needling of the skin.
3. Acne scarring—the skin becomes thicker and the results are superior to dermabrasion.
4. To tighten skin after liposuction.
5. Stretch marks (Fig. 5).
6. Lax skin on the arms (Fig. 6) and abdomen (Fig. 7).
7. Scars—if they are white, then they can become more skin colored.
8. Hypertrophic burn scars—PCI can safely be used in children and may avoid procedures to release contractures.

Contraindications for percutaneous collagen induction

1. Patients who have not pretreated their skin with vitamin A.
2. Presence of skin cancers, warts, solar keratoses, or any skin infection. The needles may disseminate abnormal cells by implantation.
3. Active acne or herpes labialis infections in the face or impetigo lesions anywhere on the body.
4. Patients on any anticoagulant therapy like warfarin, heparin, and other oral anticoagulants. The presence of these drugs may cause excessive, uncontrolled bleeding. Patients previously on such treatment should have their coagulation status checked before the treatment to confirm that they have a normal clotting/bleeding profile.
5. Many patients take aspirin daily for medical or health reasons. The aspirin should be stopped at least 3 days before the procedure.
6. Allergy to local anesthetic agents or general anesthesia. These patients should be assessed by a specialist anesthetist before treatment.
7. Patients on chemotherapy, high doses of corticosteroids, or radiotherapy.
8. Patients with uncontrolled diabetes mellitus.
9. Patients with an extremely rare but severe form of keloid scarring in which virtually every pinprick becomes a keloid. Patients often have keloids on the palms of the hands or soles of the feet.

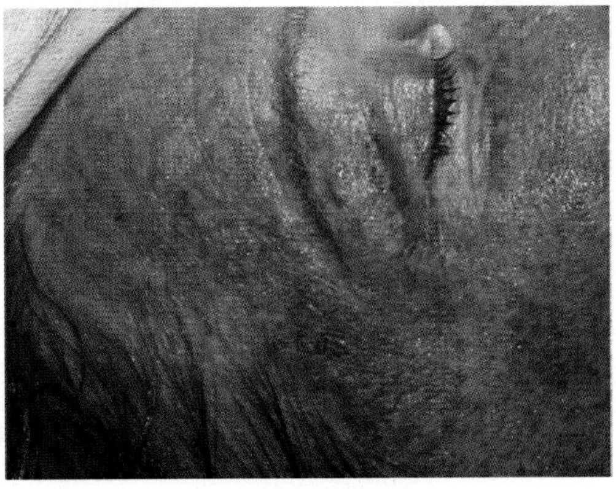

Fig. 4. Appearance of the skin immediately after PCI. The skin has been cleaned thoroughly and areas of cyanosis can be seen.

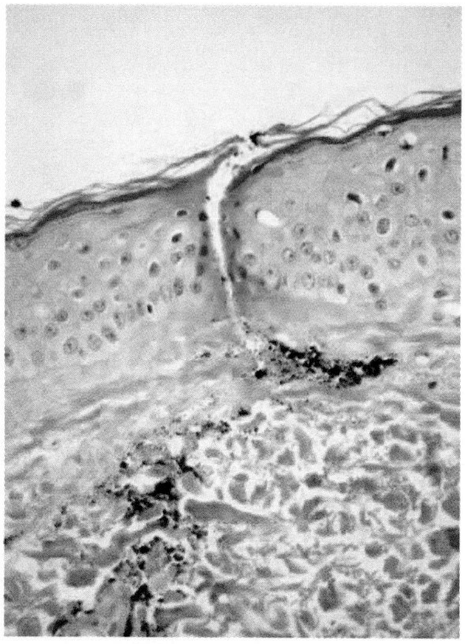

Fig. 5. This slide illustrates the ease with which Indian ink passively penetrates the skin after needling. Skin was removed from the upper eyelid and then later needled. Following needling, Indian ink was applied to the surface and allowed to dry before the specimen was placed in formalin for histologic examination. Notice that the ink has penetrated the papillary dermis. The lesson from this procedure is that clinicians and patients must be cautious about what is applied to the surface of the skin after needling.

Preparing the skin

To achieve youthful skin, one needs the skin to be functionally as young as possible. Most patients coming for rejuvenation have photoaging and this needs to be addressed before attempting any PCI. Photoaging not only is due to the actual ultraviolet damage of dermal tissues but also is the result of a chronic deficiency of vitamin A. [5] The first step toward skin health is to topically replace photosensitive vitamin A [6] and the other antioxidants vitamins C and E and carotenoids, which are normally lost on exposure to light. Vitamin A is utterly essential for the normal physiology of skin and yet it is destroyed by exposure to light so that it is prevented from exerting its important influence on skin and preserving collagen. Vitamin A is believed to control between 350 to 1000 genes that control normal function, proliferation, and differentiation of cells. One cannot exaggerate the value of vitamin A in a rejuvenation program for skin, especially with PCI, because in this case, we are specifically trying to stimulate cells to induce collagen to their maximum. Vitamin A in physiologic doses will stimulate cell growth, the release of growth factors, angiogenesis [7], and the production of healthy new collagen. The DNA effects of vitamin A interact in parallel with the growth factors released by PCI. Adequate nourishment of the skin with vitamin A (not necessarily as

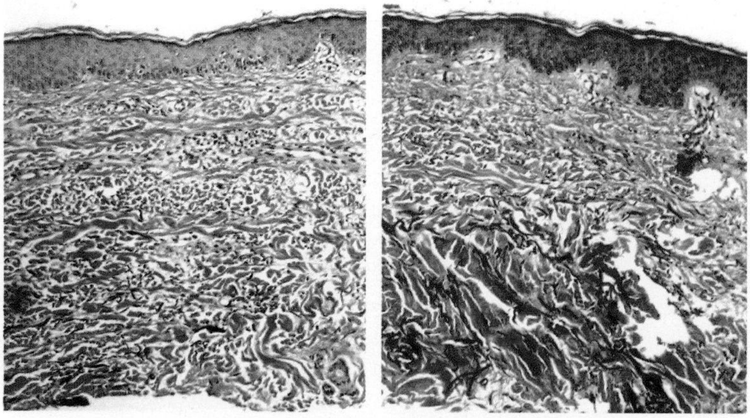

Fig. 6. (*Left image*) Histology shows thigh skin before PCI. (*Right image*) Six months after PCI, more collagen (*pink*) and elastin (*brown*) can be detected. Although difficult to estimate, there is at least 400% more collagen and elastin in the postprocedure histology section (Giemsa, original magnification × 40).

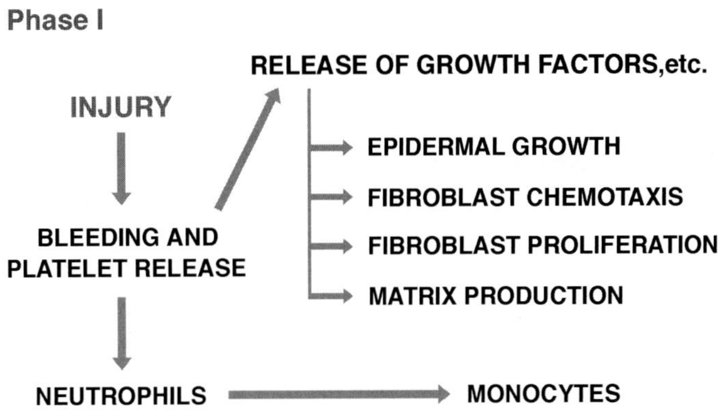

Fig. 7. Phase I of the inflammatory response showing the cascade of cytokines and growth factors following the initial injury of needling. At this stage, neutrophils are the dominant leucocytes but are gradually replaced by monocytes, the dominant leucocytes in phase II.

retinoic acid but also as retinyl esters, retinal, or retinaldehyde) will ensure that the metabolic processes for collagen production will be maximized and the skin will heal as rapidly as possible [8].

Vitamin C is similarly important for collagen formation but is destroyed by exposure to blue light. Both of these vitamins need to be replaced every day so that the natural protection and repair of DNA can be maintained. As a result, the skin will take on a more youthful appearance. The addition of palmitoyl pentapeptide or other similar peptides also will ensure that better collagen will be formed. The use of a special device for microneedling of the skin (Environ *Cosmetic* Roll-Cit, Vivida c.c., Cape Town, South Africa) will ensure that higher doses of the active ingredients get into the skin. These chemicals, however, cannot achieve really youthful skin because the collagen immediately below the epidermis has been destroyed by years of sun exposure and the production of collagen in this area needs to be stimulated by a more targeted technique.

Technique of percutaneous collagen induction

The skin is routinely prepared by using topical vitamin A and C and antioxidants for at least 3 weeks, but preferably for 3 months if the skin is very sun damaged. If the stratum corneum is thickened and rough, a series of mild TCA peels (2.5%–5% TCA in a special gel formulation) will get the surface of the skin prepared for needling and maximize the result.

Under topical, local, or general anesthesia, the skin is closely punctured with the special tool that consists of a rolling barrel with needles at regular intervals. By rolling backward and forward with

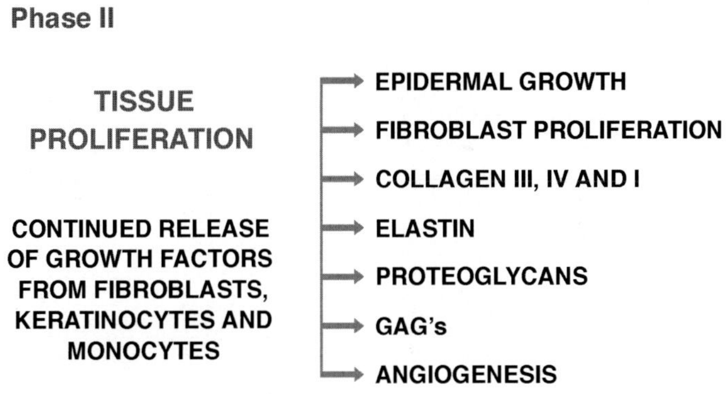

Fig. 8. Phase II of the inflammatory response, which is predominantly the stage of tissue proliferation. Monocytes, keratinocytes, and fibroblasts continue to influence and be influenced by the release of growth factors. Keratinocytes stimulate growth of the epidermis and release growth factors to promote collagen deposition by the fibroblasts. New blood vessels are created, and there is a surge of matrix deposition. GAGs, glycosaminoglycans.

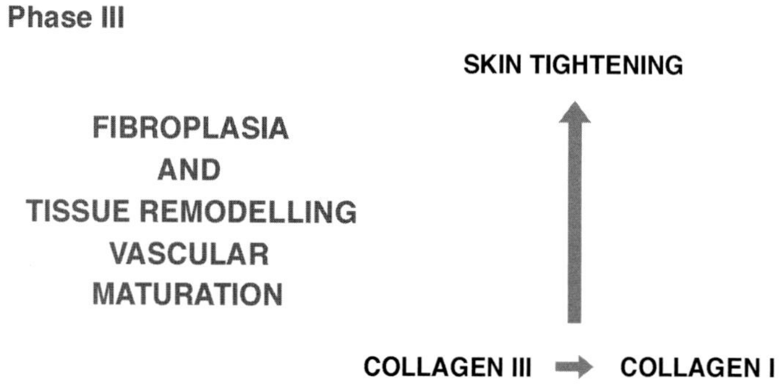

Fig. 9. The final remodeling phase of healing after PCI, which takes many months. Collagen type III is converted into collagen type I, and the skin becomes tighter. Blood supply is normalized, so the skin becomes smoother and has a natural color.

some pressure in various directions one can achieve an even distribution of the holes. The skin should be needled as densely as possible. Usually, as the needle holes get too close to each other, the needle "slips" into an established hole and so it seems impossible to over treat the skin. For very superficial small scars, I use a simple tattoo-artist's gun as described by Camirand and Doucet [3]. When using the tattoo-artist's machine, one has to be very careful not to overtreat an area because the skin can then be damaged because the needles plough their way through the skin and may remove the epidermis. The needles penetrate through the epidermis (Fig. 8) but do not remove it, so the epidermis is only punctured and will rapidly heal. The needle seems to divide cells from each other rather than cutting through the cells so that many cells are spared. Because the needles are set in a roller, the needle initially penetrates at an angle and then goes deeper as the roller turns. Finally the needle is extracted at the converse angle and therefore the tracts are curved, reflecting the path of the needle as it rolls into and then out of the skin. The epidermis and particularly the stratum corneum remain intact, except for these tiny holes, which are about four cells in diameter. The needles penetrate about 1.5 to 2 mm into the dermis (Fig. 9). Naturally, the skin bleeds for a short time, but that soon stops. The skin develops multiple microbruises in the dermis that initiate the complex cascade of growth factors that eventually results in collagen production (Fig. 10). After the bleeding stops, there is a serous ooze that has to be removed from the surface of the skin. Wet gauze swabs soak up most of the serous ooze. As the skin swells, the holes are closed, the edges of the epidermis are approximated, and the ooze stops. Noxious chemicals, however, may still penetrate the skin, so only safe molecules should be used topically (Fig. 11). After this serous leak has stopped, the skin is washed thoroughly and then covered with vitamin A, C, and

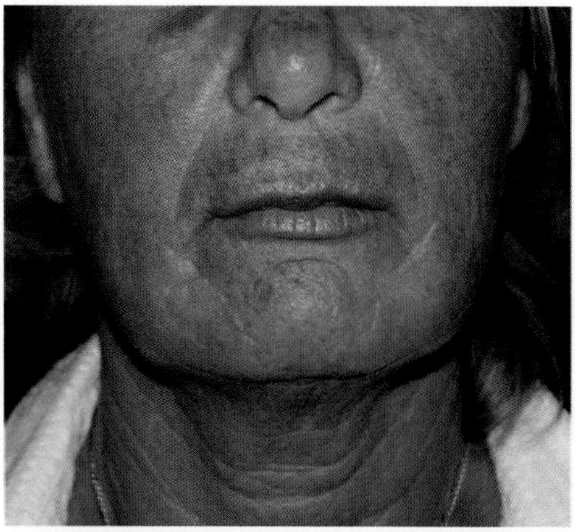

Fig. 10. Appearance of the skin 2 days after PCI.

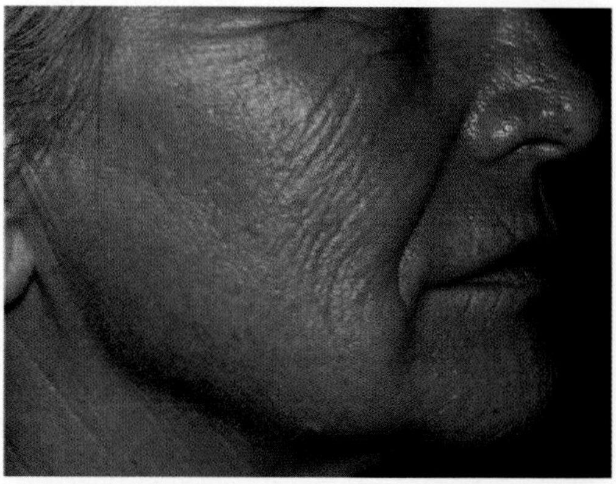

Fig. 11. Appearance of the skin 5 days after PCI. Makeup can be used from about the fourth to the fifth day without problems.

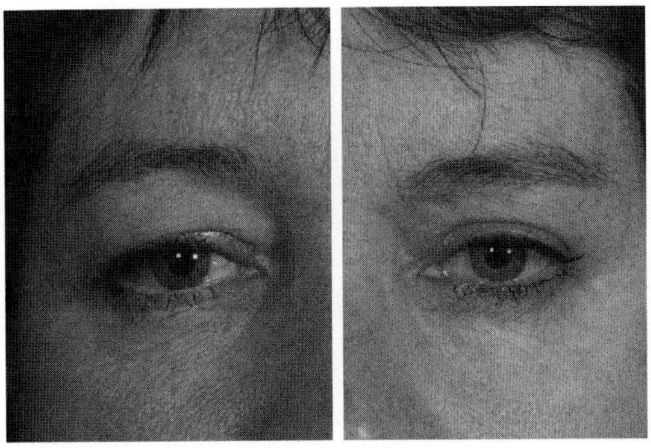

Fig. 12. Mirror image of the right eye of a patient who had PCI of the lower-eyelid skin done in conjunction with an upper blepharoplasty and lateral elevation of the eyebrow in a scarless technique devised by the author. The left image shows the right eyelid preoperatively and the right image shows the eyelid 6 months postoperatively.

E oil or cream (do not use ascorbic acid). The patient is warned that they will look terribly red and bruised, and they are encouraged to shower within a few hours of the procedure, when they return home.

Why percutaneous collagen induction works

PCI results from the natural response to wounding of the skin, even though the wound is minute and mainly subcutaneous. A single needle prick through the skin would cause an invisible response. It is necessary to understand that when the needle penetrates into the skin, this injury, minute as it might seem, causes some localized damage and bleeding by rupturing fine blood vessels. Platelets are automatically released and the normal process of inflammation commences, even though the wound is miniscule. A completely different picture emerges when thousands or tens of thousands of fine pricks are placed close to each other and one gets a field effect, because the bleeding is virtually confluent. This promotes the normal post-traumatic release of growth factors and infiltration of fibroblasts. This reaction is automatic and produces a surge of activity that inevitably leads to the fibroblasts being "instructed" to produce more collagen and elastin. The collagen is laid down in the upper dermis just below the basal layer of the epidermis (Fig. 12).

It now becomes important to understand the process of inflammation in detail. An excellent reference on this topic is the chapter "Wound Healing" by Falabela and Falanga in *The Biology of the Skin* [9]. There are three phases in wound healing:

Phase I: inflammation, which starts immediately after the injury
Phase II: proliferation (tissue formation), which starts after about 5 days and lasts about 8 weeks
Phase III: tissue remodeling, from 8 weeks to about 1 year

Phase I: initial injury

The inflammation phase starts when the needles prick the skin and rupture blood vessels and blood cells and serum gets into the surrounding tissue (Fig. 13). Platelets are important in causing clotting and releasing chemotactic factors, which cause an invasion of other platelets, leucocytes, and fibroblasts. The leucocytes, particularly neutrophils, then act on the damaged tissue to remove debris and kill bacteria. After the platelets have been activated by exposure to thrombin and collagen, they release numerous cytokines. This process involves a complex

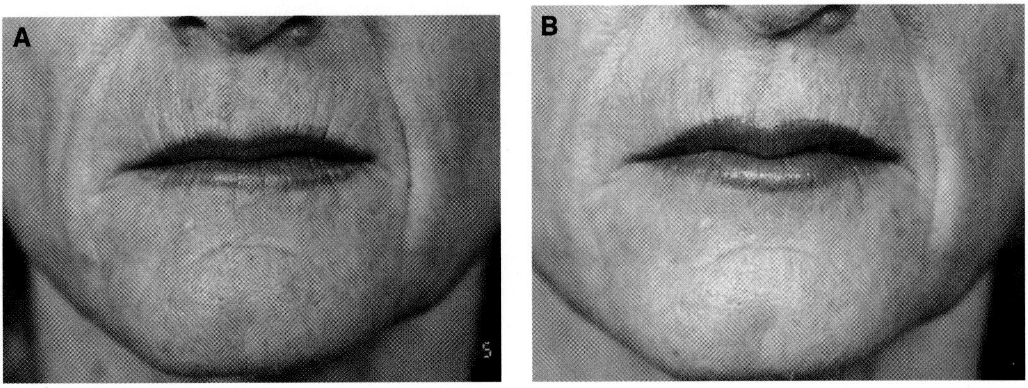

Fig. 13. (*A*) Upper lip before PCI showing lipstick tracking up the creases. (*B*) Fourteen months after one PCI treatment. No fillers have been used.

concatenation of numerous factors that are important in (1) controlling the formation of a clot (eg, fibrinogen, fibronectin, von Willebrand factor, thrombospondin, ADP, and thromboxane); (2) increasing vascular permeability, which then allows the neutrophils to pass through the vessel walls and enter the damaged area; (3) attracting neutrophils and monocytes; and (4) recruiting fibroblasts into the wounded area.

Of special interest in understanding the action of PCI are the following:

1. Fibroblast growth factor: promotes not only fibroblast proliferation but also epidermal proliferation and stimulates the production of new blood vessels. Vitamin A is an essential regulator of differentiation of fibroblasts and keratinocytes so adequate doses in the tissues are required at this stage. In anticipation of the interrupted blood supply, it should be ensured that the highest-possible normal levels of vitamin A are stored in the skin before PCI.
2. Platelet-derived growth factor: chemotactic for fibroblasts and promotes their proliferation, meaning that more collagen and elastin will be made. The need for vitamin C at this stage becomes crucial because without adequate levels of this vitamin, proline and lysine cannot be incorporated into collagen and the strands will then be defective.
3. Transforming growth factor α (TGF-α): facilitates re-epithelialization. In the case of PCI, re-epithelialization is not an important action.
4. Transforming growth factor β (TGF-β): a powerful chemotactic agent for fibroblasts that migrate into the wound about 48 hours after injury and start producing collagen types I and III, elastin, glycoseaminoglycans, and proteoglycans. Collagen type III is the dominant form of collagen in the early wound-healing phase. Again, this action is heavily dependent on adequate doses of vitamin C. At the same time, TGF-β inhibits proteases that break down the intercellular matrix.
5. Connective tissue activating peptide III: also promotes the production of intercellular matrix. Fibroblasts migrate into the area, and this surge of activity inevitably leads to the production of more collagen and more elastin. Vitamin A and C again are important mediators of this action.
6. Neutrophil activating peptide-2: has a chemotactic effect for neutrophils that then migrate into the wounded area. Neutrophils are important for killing bacteria and helping to debride tissue but, in the case of PCI, their main action is the release of cytokines that enhance the effects of the platelet cytokines (eg, platelet-derived growth factor and connective tissue growth factor).

Phase II: the period for tissue proliferation

As time passes, probably about 5 days in the case of PCI, neutrophils are replaced by monocytes (Fig. 14). The monocytes differentiate into macrophages and phagocytose the decaying neutrophils. They are very important for the later healing phases because they remove cellular debris and release several growth factors including platelet-derived growth factor, fibroblast growth factor, TGF-β, and TGF-α, which stimulate the migration and proliferation of fibroblasts and the production and modulation of extracellular matrix. With PCI, there is only extravasated blood and very little connective tissue damage to be dealt with. Bacterial infection is rare, but it has been noticed that when the needled area gets infected, greater smoothing of skin may occur, probably due to a heightened growth factor response.

In standard wounds, the inflammatory phase ends after about 5 to 6 days, as proliferation and tissue formation ensue. In these cases, the main cell is the keratinocyte. Keratinocytes change in morphology and become mobile to cover the gap in the basement membrane. The changes include retraction of tonofilaments and the dissolution of desmosomes and hemidesmosomes so that the cells can migrate. Peripheral cytoplasmic actin filaments also are developed that "pull" keratinocytes together to close the wound. These actin filaments, however, are not an important factor in PCI because re-epithelialization, or the closure of the needle holes, occurs within a few hours after needling because the gap is so small. Disruption of the basement membrane by PCI destroys the lamina lucida and brings basal keratinocytes into direct contact with the underlying collagen, which inactivates laminin and stimulates keratinocyte migration. When the keratinocytes have joined together, they start producing all the components to re-establish the basement membrane with laminin and collagen types IV and VII. A day or two after PCI, the keratinocytes start proliferating and act more in thickening the epidermis than in closing the defect.

Initially after PCI, the disruption of the blood vessels causes a moderate amount of hypoxia. The low oxygen tension stimulates the fibroblast to produce more TGF-β, platelet-derived growth factor, and endothelial growth factor. Procollagen mRNA

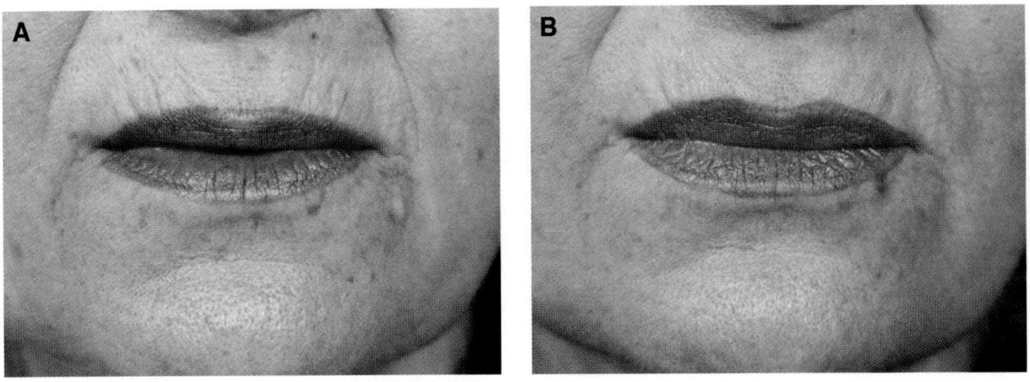

Fig. 14. (*A*) Before PCI. (*B*) One year after treatment of PCI.

also is upregulated, but this cannot cause collagen formation because oxygen is required (which only occurs when re-vascularization occurs). Collagen type III is the dominant form of collagen in the early wound-healing phase and becomes maximal 5 to 7 days after injury. The longer the initial phase, the greater the production of collagen type III.

If the injury extends deeper than the adnexal structures, then myofibroblasts may contract the wound considerably. Although the injury in skin needling extends deeper than the adnexal structures, because the epithelial wounds are simply cleft, myofibroblast wound contraction may not play a part in the healing.

A number of proteins and enzymes are important for fibroplasia and angiogenesis that develop at the same time. Anoxia, TGF-β, and fibroblast growth factor and other growth factors play an important part in angiogenesis. Fibroblasts release insulinlike growth factor that is an important stimulant for proliferation of fibroblasts themselves and endothelial cells. Insulinlike growth factor is essential in neo-vascularisation. Insulinlike growth factor or somatomedin-C also is one of the main active agents for growth hormone.

Integrins facilitate the interaction of the fibroblasts, endothelial cells, and keratinocytes.

Phase III – the process of tissue remodeling

Tissue remodeling continues for months after the injury and is mainly done by the fibroblasts (Fig. 15). By the fifth day after injury, the fibronectin matrix is laid down along the axis in which fibroblasts are aligned and in which collagen will be laid down. TGF-β and other growth factors play an important part in the formation of this matrix. Collagen type III is laid down in the upper dermis just below the basal layer of the epidermis.

Collagen type III is gradually replaced by collagen type I over a period of a year or more, which gives increased tensile strength. The matrix metalloproteinases (MMPs) are essential for the conversion process. The various MMPs are generally

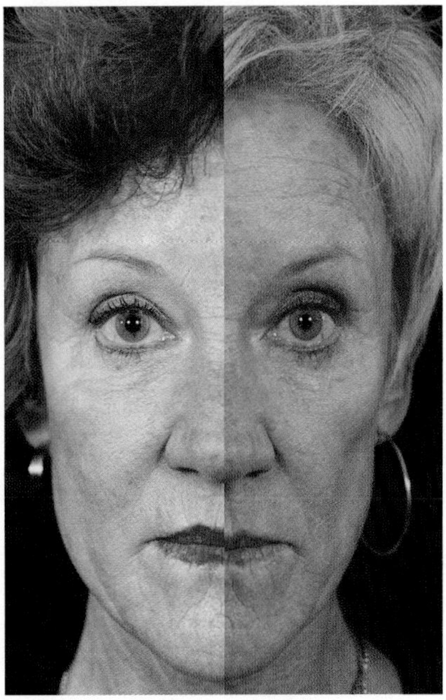

Fig. 15. Mirror image of the right side of the face preoperatively (*left image*) and 4 months after whole face needling (*right image*). The upper lip was initially needled three times 2 years before, at monthly intervals. The lower eyelid has been needled only once.

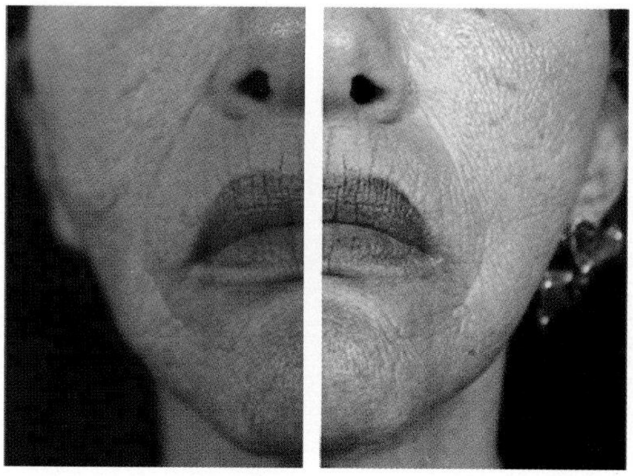

Fig. 16. Mirror image of the right side of the face of a patient previously treated with extensive silicon injections that resulted in terrible wrinkling and sagging of her facial skin. This wrinkling and sagging had improved with suction aspiration and a face-lift. (*Left image*) One year after the face-lift. The skin is still terribly wrinkled and sagging. (*Right image*) The patient 1 year after PCI of the whole face and a scarless malar lift without any skin excision.

classed as MMP-1 (collagenases), MMP-2 (gelatinases), and MMP-3 (stromelysins).

Care of the skin after percutaneous collagen induction

Immediately after the treatment, the skin looks bruised, but bleeding is minimal and there is only a small ooze of serum that soon stops. The author recommends soaking the skin with saline swabs for an hour or two and then cleaning the skin thoroughly with a Tea Tree Oil–based cleanser. The patient is encouraged to use topical vitamin A and vitamin C as a cream or an oil to promote better healing and greater production of collagen. The addition of peptides like palmitoyl pentapeptide could possibly ensure even better results.

At home, the patient should stand under a shower for a long time, allowing the water to soak into the surface of the skin. Bathing is discouraged because of potential contamination from drains and plugs. Patients should be reminded to use only tepid water because the skin will be more sensitive to heat. While the water is running over the face or body, the patient should gently massage the treated skin until all serum, blood, or oil is removed. The importance of a thorough but gentle washing of the skin, a few hours after the procedure, cannot be stressed enough.

The skin will feel tight and may look uncomfortable in a few cases. Most patients say that the skin is a little sensitive but the major complaint is about the bruising and swelling. The following day, the skin looks less dramatic (Fig. 16) and by day 4 or 5, the skin has returned to a moderate pink flush, which can easily be concealed with makeup (Fig. 17). Men usually seem to heal faster and are less bruised than women. From day 3 or 4 onward, iontophoresis [10] and low-frequency sonophoresis of vitamin A and C could maximize the induction of healthy collagen. Iontophoresis also tends to reduce the swelling of the skin, which also helps the patient look better sooner. Low-frequency sonophoresis can be used alone without iontophoresis to enhance penetration of palmitoyl pentapeptide or other peptides (eg, palmitoyl hexapeptide, copper peptides, and so forth), which also may increase the creation of healthy collagen and elastin.

After the skin has been needled, it becomes easier to penetrate, and much higher doses of vitamin A become available in the depth of the skin. Higher doses of vitamin A may cause a retinoid reaction

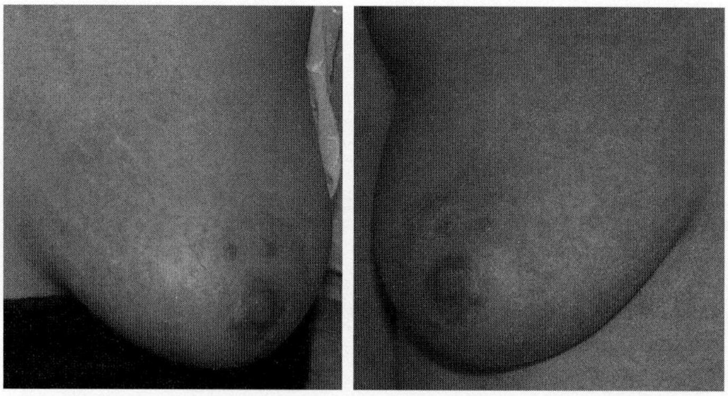

Fig. 17. Mirror image of the right breast to show stretch marks before PCI (*left image*) and 6 months after PCI (*right image*). The stretch marks have become virtually invisible.

even though the milder forms of vitamin A (eg, retinyl palmitate) are being used. This reaction will aggravate the pink flush of the skin and also cause dry, flaky skin. Needling may cause some slight roughness of the skin surface for a few days, and this condition is definitely worse when topical vitamin A is used. The clinician should ignore this and urge the patient to continue using the topical vitamin A. Patients usually anticipate that their skin will get red and do not complain much about that but become concerned about the dryness. It should be remembered that the skin has lost the important barrier function of keeping the water inside the skin. Until this barrier function is restored completely after a few days, the skin will feel dry. A hydrating cream or even petrolatum can be used to soothe the dry sensation.

When the patient has not cleaned the skin thoroughly, a fine scab may form on the surface. The formation of scabs should be discouraged because they may cause obstruction and the development of simple milia or tiny pustules. Milia are uncommon but when they occur, they should be treated by pricking and draining. Tiny pustules are more common and usually found in patients treated for acne scars. It is important to open them early and make sure that the skin has been cleaned thoroughly and that there is no serous residue on the surface. When the pustules are allowed to dry on the skin, they will form thin scabs that effectively prevent the penetration of the vitamins necessary for a successful treatment.

The patient should avoid direct sun exposure for at least 10 days if possible and use a broad-brimmed hat or scarf to protect the facial skin.

Patients may shocked when they look in the mirror, but this procedure is a far less shocking experience than laser resurfacing.

The treatment can be repeated a month later, but the best interval between treatments is presently unknown. If a clinician intends to achieve a smoothing comparable to a laser resurfacing, then depending on the original state, a patient may require three or even four treatments. The results that are achieved are not temporary but endure for many years. Again, it should be emphasized that this progress is utterly dependent on adequate nutrition for the skin.

Predicted appearance after percutaneous collagen induction

1. Immediately after procedure: bleeding and bruising
2. Five to 20 minutes after procedure: bleeding stops quickly; serum oozes from the skin
3. Day 1: bruised and dark purple-red appearance in light skin; puffy facial appearance; some bruising, especially close to eyes and in thin-skinned areas
4. Day 2: red-purple hue on light skin like a moderate sun burn; bruising, if any, starts to lighten; swelling may be worse on the second day in many people, and most people are not ready to be seen in public at this stage
5. Day 3: appearance still pink, with bruising getting steadily lighter; swelling reduced; some people ready to appear in public but could be conspicuous
6. Day 4 to 6: minimal swelling; bruising will take a few days to disappear; can use makeup; patient can appear in public with confidence with the use of makeup
7. Day 7: in most patients, very few signs are visible of the procedure. Most patients should be advised to stay off work for between 5 and10 days if they deal with people at work and are sensitive about their own appearance

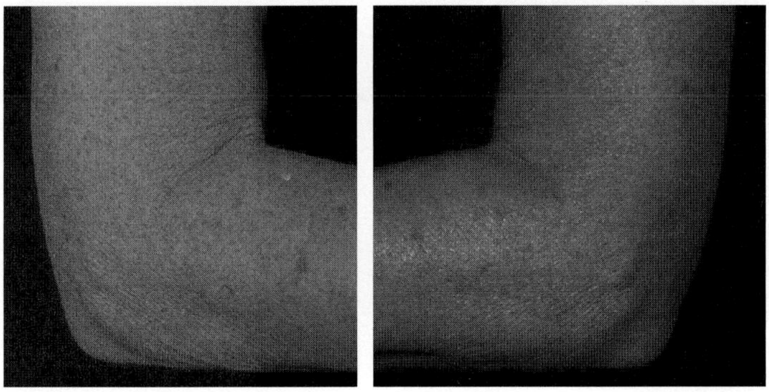

Fig. 18. Mirror image of the right arm shows wrinkling and loose skin prior to PCI (*left image*) and tighter skin 4 months after one session of PCI (*right image*).

Note about darker, pigmented skin

Most patients with dark, type IV and V skin will not show the amount of bruising that Medical Roll-Cit usually causes. The skin will appear puffy, and bruising might be visible only in thin-skinned areas such as around the eyes. Changes are a lot less visible than in light-skinned individuals. Darker-skinned patients should protect the skin from exposure to sunlight and, if necessary, a zinc oxide paste should be used to ensure ultraviolet light protection. A complication many people fear is the risk of hyperpigmentation. Tattoos are rarely hyperpigmented, even in darker-skinned people. The author has never seen hyperpigmentation in patients with darker skins (eg, African, Indian, Malaysian, Chinese, Mediterranean) that have been needled.

Results of percutaneous collagen induction

PCI has been used with success for lower-eyelid wrinkles (see Fig. 2), upper-lip lines (see Figs. 3 and 4), facial wrinkles (see Fig. 5; Fig. 18), and lax photo-damaged skin on the arms (see Fig. 7), abdomen (Fig. 19), and legs. It is also useful for reducing the appearance of stretch marks (see Fig. 6) so that they become almost invisible. It is particularly useful for acne scars and post burn scars. The scars will flatten and, after a few treatments, the mesh marks of skin grafts will be less obvious.

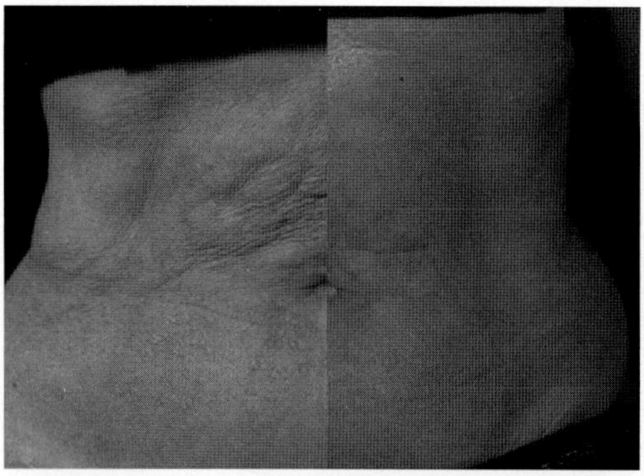

Fig. 19. Mirror image of the right side of the abdomen before PCI (*left image*) and 4 months after PCI (*right image*) showing smoothening of the abdominal skin. A second session of PCI will smoothen the redundant skin.

Advantages of percutaneous collagen induction

1. PCI does not damage the skin. Histology has shown that the skin is indistinguishable from normal skin and that the epidermis may show more dermal papillae.
2. Skin becomes thicker, with greater than a 400% increase in collagen deposition and significantly more elastin (Fig. 6).
3. Any part of the body may be treated.
4. The healing phase is short.
5. Compared with laser resurfacing, it is less expensive and the skin is healthier.
6. May be safely done in people with darker pigmented skin, without fear of hyperpigmentation.
7. The skin does not become sun sensitive.
8. Can be done on people who have had laser resurfacing or have very thin skin.
9. Telangiectasia generally improves probably because the vessels are ruptured in so many places that they cannot be repaired.
10. The technique is easy to master using a new tool that has been specially designed for the procedure and does not necessarily have to be done by a plastic surgeon or dermatologist.
11. PCI can even be done using topical anesthesia for limited areas.

Disadvantages of percutaneous collagen induction

1. Exposure to blood. This procedure is relatively bloody, much the same as dermabrasion.
2. Although PCI cannot achieve as intense a deposition of collagen as laser resurfacing, the treatment can be repeated to get even better results that will last as long if not longer than laser resurfacing.
3. Overaggressive needling may cause scarring, particularly when using a tattoo gun. This scarring does not seem to occur when using the special barrel of needles.
4. Herpes simplex is an uncommon complication and patients are instructed to use a topical virocidal if they feel the tingling feeling typical of herpes.

Summary

PCI is a simple technique and, with the right tool, can thoroughly puncture any skin easily and quickly. Although a single treatment may not give the smoothing that is seen with laser resurfacing, the epidermis remains virtually normal. When the result is not sufficient, treatment can be repeated. The technique can be used on areas that are not suitable for peeling or laser resurfacing.

References

[1] Orentreich DS, Orentreich N. Subcutaneous incisionless (subcision) surgery for the correction of depressed scars and wrinkles. Dermatol Surg 1995;21(6):543–9.
[2] Fernandes D. Upper lip line treatment. Paper presented at the ISAPS Conference. Taipei, Taiwan, October 1996.
[3] Camirand A, Doucet J. Needle dermabrasion. Aesth Plast Surg 1997;21(1):48–51.
[4] Fernandes D. Skin needling as an alternative to laser. Paper presented at the IPRAS Conference, San Francisco, CA, June 1999.
[5] Fisher GJ, Wang ZQ, Datta SC, et al. Pathophysiology of premature skin aging induced by ultraviolet light. N Engl J Med 1997;337(20):1419–28.
[6] Fisher GJ, Datta SC, Talwar HS, et al. Molecular basis of sun-induced premature skin aging and retinoid antagonism. Nature 1996;379(6563):335–9.
[7] Diaz BV, Lenoir MC, Ladoux A, et al. Regulation of vascular endothelial growth factor expression in human keratinocytes by retinoids. J Biol Chem 2000; 275(1):642–50.
[8] Varani J, Fisher GJ, Kang S, et al. Molecular mechanisms of intrinsic skin aging and retinoid-induced repair and reversal. J Investig Dermatol Symp Proc 1998;3(1):57–60.
[9] Falabella AF, Falanga V. Wound healing. In: Freinkel RK, Woodley DT, editors. The biology of the skin. New York: Parthenon Publishing Group; 2001. p. 281–97.
[10] Schmidt JB, Binder M, Macheiner W, et al. New treatment of atrophic acne scars by iontophoresis with estriol and tretinoin. Int J Dermatol 1995;34(1):53–7.

ELSEVIER
SAUNDERS

Oral Maxillofacial Surg Clin N Am 17 (2005) 65 – 76

ORAL AND MAXILLOFACIAL SURGERY CLINICS of North America

Suture Suspension Lifts: A Review

John Flynn, MB BS, Dip Obst RACOG, FRACGP, Dip P Derm, FACCS

Cosmedic Clinic, Level I, Ashmore Medical Centre, Ashmore, PO Box 567, Ashmore City, Gold Coast 4214, Australia

There has been a recent trend toward minimally invasive procedures in all facets of cosmetic surgery. This trend is in keeping with a general movement toward more effective procedures with less tissue injury and less downtime for the patient. The hope, of course, is that this trend translates to happier patients with fewer complications. An area where this aim is keenly felt is in facial rejuvenation. Our face is the self-portrait we show to the world; we want to present it in a good light, and there is a never-ending stimulus to present it well. Society's attitudes toward aging seem to have changed considerably over the past several generations, and although we have generally agreed and reluctantly accepted that we cannot stop aging, we do not necessarily need to show its full effects.

This change of community attitudes is an important stimulus for the development and popularity of suture suspension techniques. We live in an age of instant "on" (eg, instant coffee, instant Internet access), so why not instant "lift" and instant recovery, or at least as near to this as possible?

What defines a suture suspension technique?

All face-lifts are held in place with sutures well placed to lift, provide support for the tissues, and tighten. In short, the main characteristic that provides suture distinction is the accompanying dissection or lack thereof. Face-lifts, whether they are of a superficial musculoaponeurotic system (SMAS) elevation type, deep plane lift, or minilift, involve a degree of tissue dissection that creates a skin flap and a further SMAS advancement as an imbrication or advancement flap. These elements are then sutured in place with the edges in approximation. Numerous sutures, usually individually placed, are used to hold and support the tissues in their new position. Further, the plane of dissection results in an area of tissue that has been traumatized by the dissection and naturally proceeds to heal, producing a scar. The scar adherence occurs over a wide area, causing a side-to-side adherence that also supports the tissue in its new position (Fig. 1). The next pertinent issue is that the repair involves multiple layers of suturing and scar formation. Because it is the scar that provides the support required for longevity of the lift, dissolvable sutures may be used. In the various suture suspension techniques, it is the continued integrity of the suture that provides for the longevity of the lift; therefore, permanent sutures need to be employed.

The elements that cause bruising, swelling, and discomfort are the same elements that provide the security of the support in a surgical lift by virtue of the dissection, approximation of the tissues, and the scar formation that naturally occurs as a result of tissue injury.

Placement of any suture can be thought of as involving an anchor point, a point of purchase, and approximation of tissue. Traditional suture techniques involved in face-lifts can be thought of as bringing the anchor point and the point of purchase together. In a suture suspension technique, there is an anchor point and a point of purchase, and although there is an element of approximation, these points tend to remain separated by various distances (Fig. 2). In addition, there is generally little or no intervening scar tissue support, so the integrity of the suture material is a prime consideration.

E-mail address: drflynn@cosmedic.com.au

doi:10.1016/j.coms.2004.10.002

oralmaxsurgery.theclinics.com

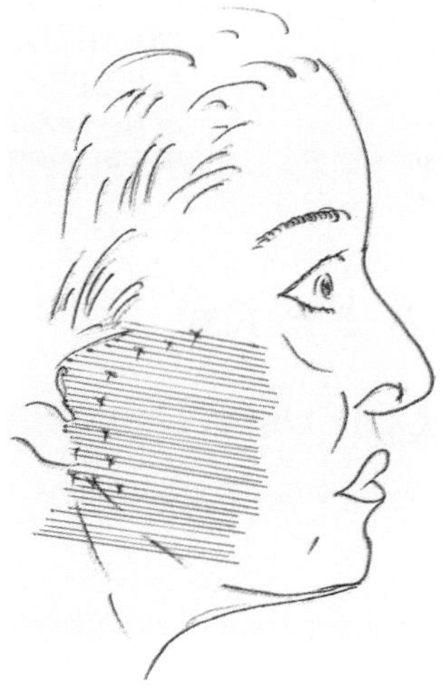

Fig. 1. Schematic depiction of line of sutures in SMAS advancement and the wide area of dissection, allowing side-to-side scar adherence and, hence, a more stable lift.

The next pertinent difference is that with the suture suspension techniques, the material is placed without significant dissection of tissues, often placed by a hollow trocar or spinal-type needle. The same features that give the suture suspension techniques some advantage insofar as less recovery time, less bruising, and fewer complications carry the disadvantages of a less stable lift and reduced longevity. Patients and many practitioners see that the advantages significantly outweigh the disadvantages. The most advantageous features are that these techniques can usually be performed in well-equipped rooms rather than hospital suites, they are quick and have fast recovery, and minor asymmetries or lack of effect can easily be remedied.

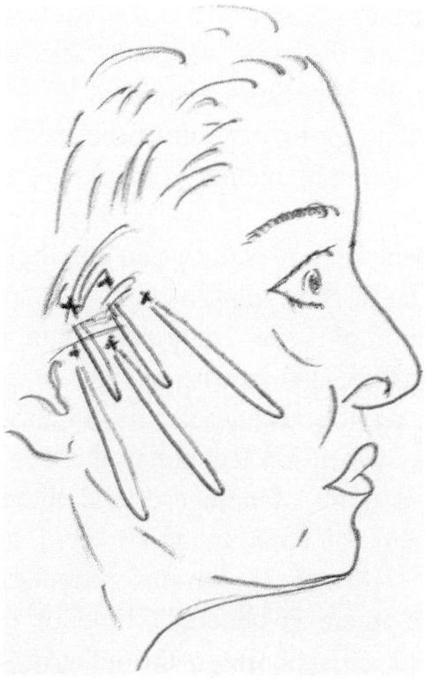

Fig. 2. Schematic depiction of loop suspension sutures as in stitch lift, with an anchor point and a point of purchase remaining at some distance from each other.

Many clinicians are familiar with the Giampappa suture [1] used to accentuate the submental angle and to support sagging neck skin. In these techniques, the suture is fixed at both ends to the mastoid fascia and the suture is strung between these two points to achieve the desired effect.

This technique represents a true suspension of the anterior neck and floor of the mouth but is not the procedure on which this article is focused. To some extent, the S-Lift [2] could be considered a suture suspension technique because of the limited dissection and the placement of the purse-string or "O" and "U" sutures to advance or "suspend" the cheek tissues.

Candidate selection

The success (or otherwise) of any technique certainly depends on proper execution of the process but probably depends more on the selection of the appropriate candidate for the procedure. Suture suspension procedures are more appropriate for a younger group of patients (35–50 years). The best candidate should require only subtle improvement and have good-quality skin and adequate facial volume. Facial lipoatrophy is a relative contraindication because the desired effect of the lift, especially in the midface, is to lift the fat pads. The presence of significant skin laxity poses a risk of redundant skin fold or "ripples" and inadequate elevation, and skin excision may be required. Although skin has some inherent retractability, there is a limit to this and, of course, it diminishes with age. Poor subcutaneous support tissue also more likely results in a "dimple" at the point of purchase.

Antiptosis suture threads

First described in 1998 by Dr. Malin Sulimanidze, a Russian surgeon, antiptosis suture (APTOS) threads have led to a renewed interest in suture suspension techniques. Sulimanidze et al [3] described a series of 157 patients between 22 and 77 years old (average, 49 years). The Web site www.aptos.ru features a series of slides depicting the APTOS technique and a number of case studies. Assessment of the photos

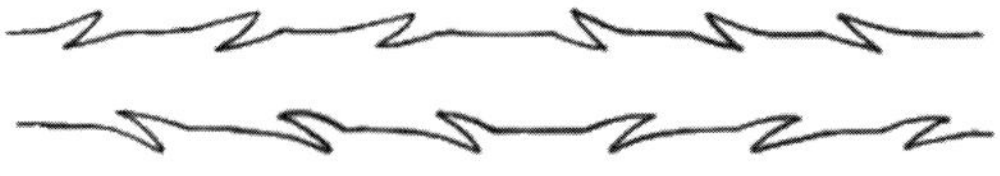

Fig. 3. Magnified depiction of a longitudinal section of APTOS thread with bilateral (converging) direction of cogs. More information can be found at the Web site www.aptos.ru (go to "New Technologies," select "APTOS," and "see slides").

of these case studies confirms the generally younger age of APTOS patients compared to the usual age group of face-lift patients.

APTOS threads are made of a polypropylene suture material, with angled cuts along the length of the thread creating barbs. These barbs can be divergent or convergent to suit the application desired (Fig. 3). Dr. Sulimanidz has lodged a patent for APTOS threads [3]. In the United States, the term *Feather Lift*, used to describe the process by which these threads are used to produce a facial lift, is trademarked by KMI (Kolster Methods Inc., Corona, CA) and Dr. Ron Fragen [4]. The Feather Lift Web site (www.featherlift.com) shows a description of the technique and lists indications including "drooping of the soft tissue of the face and neck, weakly pronounced aesthetic contours, flaccid, flat face and premature aging and sun damaged face."

Feather Lift

The Feather Lift describes the placement of APTOS threads to elevate the outer brows, malar area, jowls, and neck (Fig. 4).

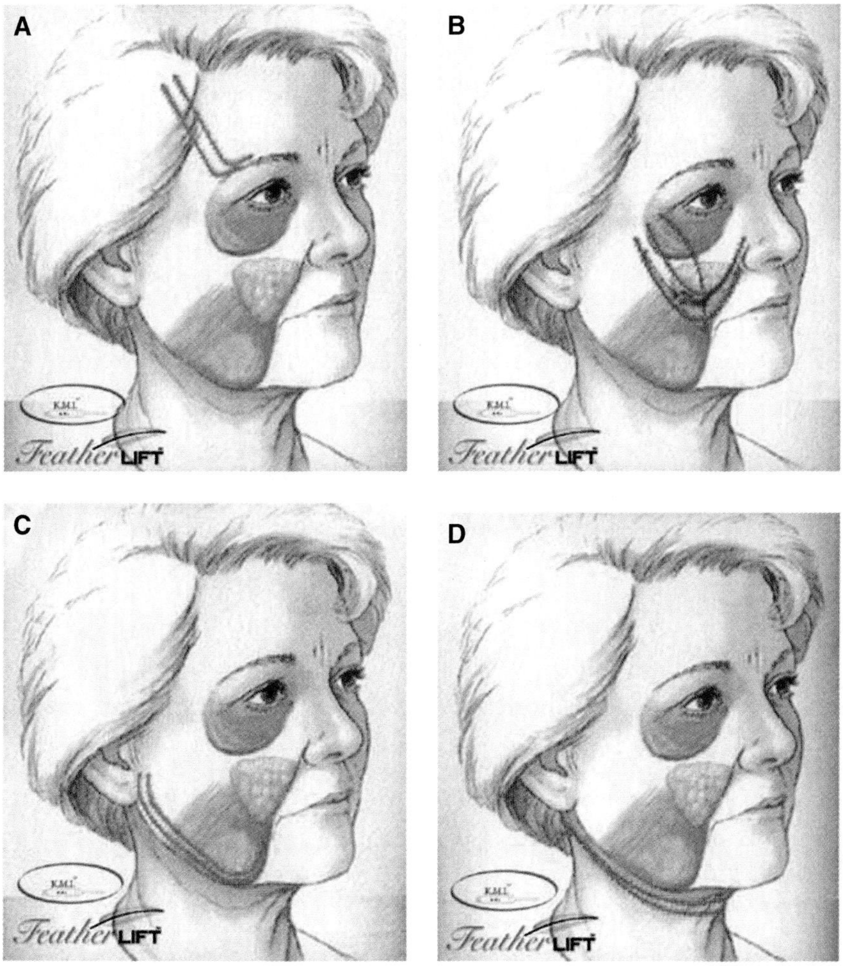

Fig. 4. Diagrams of the Feather Lift placement of APTOS threads for elevation of brow (*A*), cheek (*B*), jowls (*C*), and neck (*D*). (Courtesy of www.featherlift.com; with permission.)

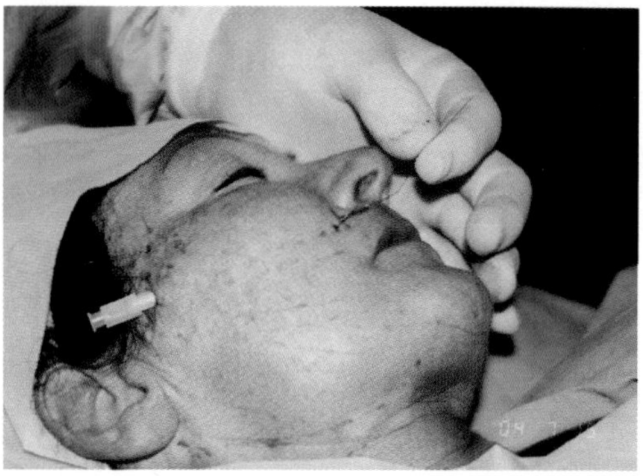

Fig. 5. Insertion of the APTOS threads by way of a spinal needle used as a trocar. Previously inserted threads are still evident. Trimming of the ends of the threads occurs after satisfactory insertion of all the threads.

After careful marking of the placement of the threads, a hollow trocar or spinal-type needle is threaded along the marked path and the APTOS thread inserted. The tissue is held and compressed to conform to the desired position and the trocar is withdrawn, leaving the APTOS in place (Fig. 5). The barbs engage the subcutaneous tissue and hold to the new position. In the usual case, the APTOS threads are of the convergent variety. In the inferior, the suture the barbs are angled cephalad. This position allows for the elevation effect of the thread. The superior segment has barbs angled caudad and forms a bolster against the tissues falling back. In a sense, the superior segment acts as an anchor point and the inferior segment acts as the point of purchase. The particular advantage is that there is a fairly broad area of contact with the threads and numerous points of engagement with the tissue to provide a good support network. One particular disadvantage is that the anchor point is somewhat floating in the subcutaneous tissue, reliant on engagement by the "cogs" rather than having a secure base.

As with any foreign object inserted into the skin, an inflammatory reaction is generated and scar tissue is formed around the thread. Because of the barbs of the APTOS thread, a firm "capture" of the thread is formed to secure its position (Fig. 6).

Stitch lift

In this process, a series of loop sutures are inserted in the subcutaneous plane to achieve elevation of tissue. One particular advantage of this method is the secure anchor point, but the disadvantage is the single purchase point at the apex of the loop, and depending on the laxity of the skin, a retraction dimple is more common. To redress this situation, the loops are inserted in a serial fashion to distribute and support the skin tension (see Fig. 2).

Again, sutures are threaded by way of a spinal needle, but in this case, the needle is left attached to the thread, which allows a bite of deeper tissue and

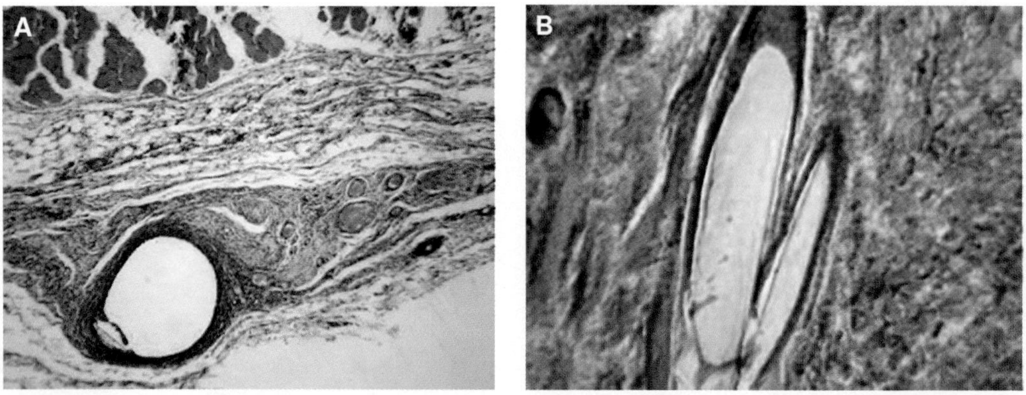

Fig. 6. (*A, B*) Histologic slides depicting APTOS threads and cogs and the inflammatory response to the threads. This inflammatory reaction results in scar formation that "captures" or "secure" the position of the thread. It is expected that the natural scar contraction should produce further support and lift over time as the scar matures. (Courtesy of Austramedex (Victoria, Australia), distributors of APTOS threads in Australia; with permission.)

knotting to provide a secure anchor point. The spinal needle pierces the skin inferiorly to form the purchase point. The needle is threaded superiorly (or supero-laterally, as the case may be) in the subcutaneous plane and exits by way of a stab incision usually at the hairline or within the hairline. The suture, typically a 4-0 nylon or polypropylene suture with an 18-mm needle attached is inserted from the superior end and threaded through the spinal needle. The spinal needle is withdrawn to almost the full extent and, still with the suture inside, advanced again toward the superior stab incision. The secondary course of the spinal needle is at a deeper plane to catch onto SMAS or, in the case of the brow, the frontalis. On exiting the superior wound, the running end of the suture is retrieved and thus forms a loop. With the needle still attached to the standing end, a bite of deeper tissue is taken and a knot is formed to provide fixation.

This method has good application in the brow and cheek and can also be used to tighten the loose skin of the neck.

Secure anchoring filaments for facial elevation lift

After experiencing the particular advantages and disadvantages of the stitch lift, loop-type sutures, and APTOS, the author developed an alternative suture suspension. When used in combination with other suture suspension techniques to achieve a face-lift effect, this technique has been dubbed the SAfFE (secure anchoring filaments for facial elevation) lift. With this technique, a 2-0 polypropylene suture is used and barbs are cut to an APTOS-like configuration. There is, however, a segment without barbs where the loop is formed because barbs here would weaken the thread too severely (Fig. 7). The needle remains attached, and the thread is placed in the same manner as the stitch lift.

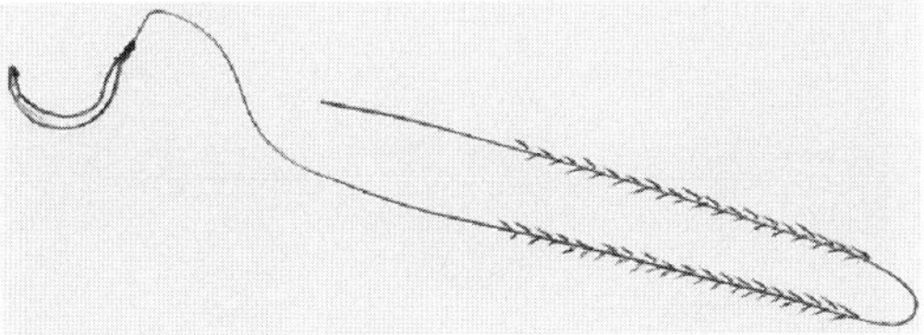

Fig. 7. Depiction of a SAfFE filament. The needle remains attached, and there are barbs with a clear segment at what would be the apex of the loop.

The advantage is having the continuous engagement of the APTOS thread with the availability of a secure anchor through a knotted bit of deeper tissue. Because of the larger gauge of thread, the knot is correspondingly larger and needs to be buried and located behind the hairline. This suture suspension is particularly good in elevating the malar pad, with fixation to the temporalis fascia above the ear.

Singapore surgeon Dr. Woffles Wu described a similar suture but without the retained needle. The fixation is achieved in the temporalis facsia with another suture (Woffles Wu, personal communication, March 2004). These threads need to be individually crafted and, at the time of this writing, are not available commercially.

One theoretic advantage of the SAfFE filament is the scar tissue response previously mentioned that locks the barbed portion of the thread in place while the smooth portion retains the ability to move within its "fibrous capsule." The body naturally forms a foreign body reaction along the whole length of the suture. The barbed portion becomes fixed because of the irregularities of the barbs but the non barbed portion forms a smooth covering which allows movement along the line of the tract. This smooth tract allows the advantage that later location of the filament near its anchor point and advancement or tightening to readjust after a period of aging and descent. Formation of scar tissue over time should act to form a permanent framework of linear scars that contract in the expected manner to maintain and even enhance the lift. It begs the question of whether the threads can be made of absorbable material and still have longevity of effect without the persistence of foreign material. First thoughts suggest that patients might find this an attractive feature. The author has approached the manufacturers of APTOS on this point and it appears to be under consideration.

Approaches for various locations

Eyebrows

Eye area rejuvenation is one of the more frequently requested procedures. Blepharoplasty is well described. Brow elevation offers a number of surgical options of varying degrees of complexity, and assessment of some suture suspension techniques is warranted. The eyebrow is a very mobile portion of the forehead that is capable of active elevation, descent, and medial movement by way of its muscular attach-

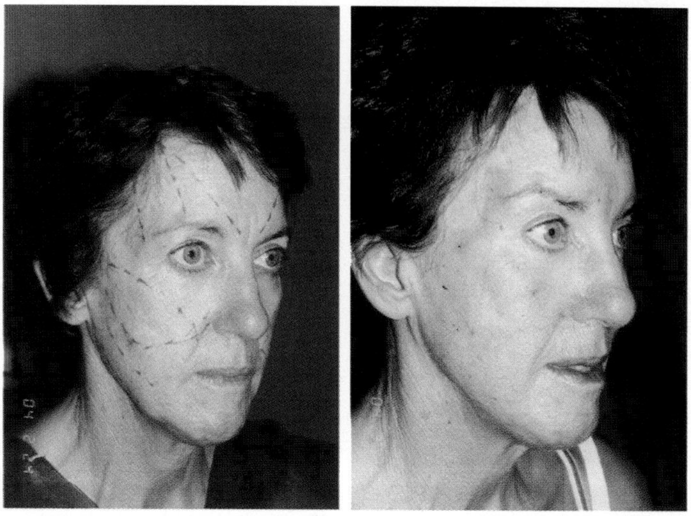

Fig. 8. Before (*left image*) and after (*right image*) loop suture suspension (stitch lift) of brow, with creation of a definite arch in the eyebrow. The more central markings relate to the positioning of APTOS threads to distract the frown lines in the glabela. The cheek markings refer to placement of APTOS for elevation of malar and SAfFE filaments for tightening the jowls. This combination of suture suspension techniques forms the basis of the SAfFE Lift approach.

ments. Elevation without skin tightening or removal needs to be subtle to avoid dimpling and prominent skin folds.

Options for elevation

The author first saw loop suture suspension for the brow described by Dr. Des Fernandes from South Africa at the annual conference of The Australasian College of Cosmetic Surgery [5].

The author has been pleased with the results using this lift. It offers the ability to shape the brow by virtue of the different placement of the sutures. Sutures can number one to four in each brow. Placement can give an even elevation, create a more defined arch, or simply raise the lateral or medial portion of the brow. There is good scope for variation to match a patient's particular desire. The end result is easily adjustable by adding or removing sutures.

Antiptosis suture

The technique described for the Feather Lift allows for some elevation, primarily of the lateral portion of the eyebrow, but also gives a superolateral vector.

Other vectors of the APTOS have been used by the author with some success (Fig. 8). In this patient, the aim was some medial elevation of the brow and some degree of distraction over the glabela to try to improve the frown lines. It should be noted that when using either suspension technique, it is helpful to use botulinum toxin in the corrugators and lateral obicularis oculi at the same time. Botulinum toxin is well known for its usefulness in brow shaping and can be used here to compliment the suture suspension. Strong activation of the brow depressors can affect the result of the suture lift in the early stages (Fig. 9). By the time the botulinum toxin has worn off after some months, the threads are well supported by

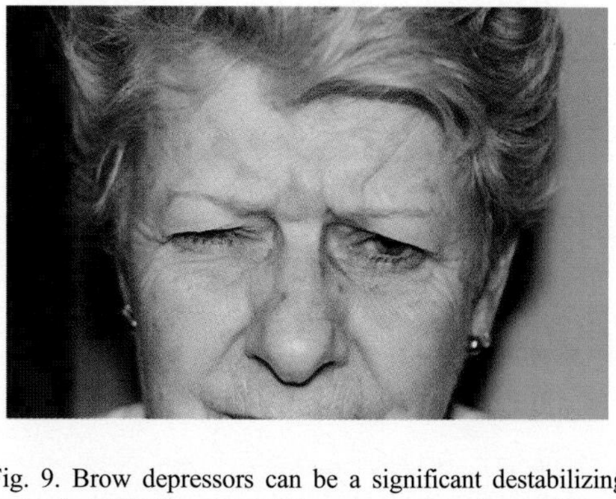

Fig. 9. Brow depressors can be a significant destabilizing factor in APTOS or stitch lift eyebrow elevation, and botulinum toxin is a useful adjunctive therapy.

the fibrous results of the inflammatory reaction that their insertion engenders.

Complications

- Palpable knots (minimized by using a 4-0 suture)
- Dimpling at entry/exit points (usually resolves spontaneously over 2–3 weeks)
- Extrusion of APTOS threads (easily trimmed)
- Bruising or black eyes (usually uncommon and small in extent)
- Prominent folds of redundant skin (should be minimal in well-selected candidates and normally resolve)

It should be noted that even though dimpling will usually resolve with little intervention, it may be distressing to patients. A small amount of a fine-textured dermal filler or polylactic acid solves the problem quickly; by the time the filler has dissipated, the dimple is fully resolved.

Malar enhancement

It is in correction of the malar fat pad that the threads are seen to best advantage. The aim is to elevate the midface and help to correct the prominence of the nasolabial folds. The technique also has the advantage of causing a "mounding" effect of the malar pad to give more prominence.

APTOS threads

The placement of the threads follows gentle curves and of the three described placements, the

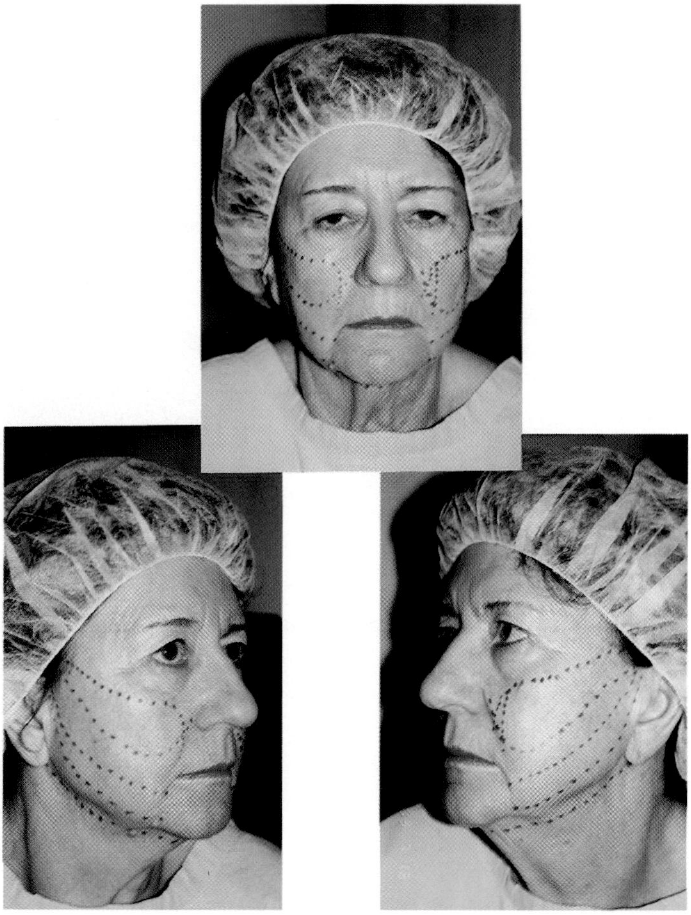

Fig. 10. Series of photos showing markings for APTOS placement that differ from those depicted in the Feather Lift.

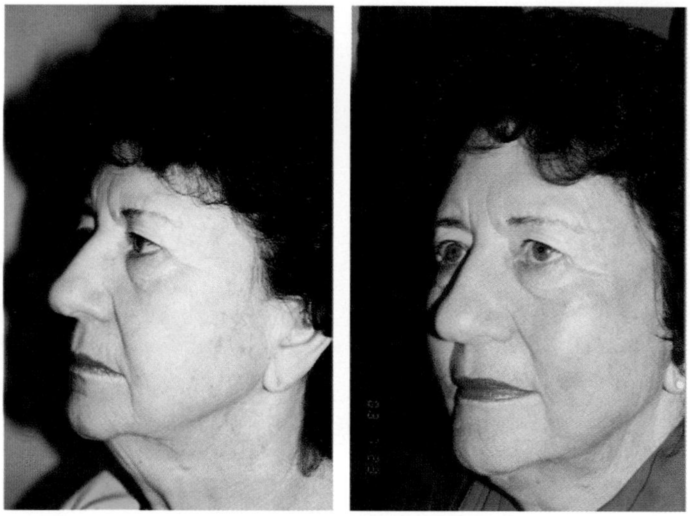

Fig. 11. Before (*left image*) and 3 days after (*right image*) insertion of APTOS threads. This patient is older than the usual candidate for this procedure. There is modest bruising, subtle but significant improvement of the jowls, and definition of the mandible. The light reflex on the malar prominence indicates the volumetric improvement of the cheek.

uppermost is designed to lift and compress the malar pad and the lower two threads are to support the lift. Different placement of the threads can alter the vectors and subtly alters the malar shift (Figs. 10 and 11).

The APTOS effect is often subtle. Alteration of the placement of the threads helps to avoid skin creases in the finer, more delicate tissue of older patients. In younger patients, there is usually seen a more significant tissue shift (Fig. 12).

Stitch lift

Sutures, usually 3-0 or 4-0 gauge, are placed serially in increasing lengths, with the temporal hairline as the exit point with fixation to the temporalis fascia. The lower fixation point should avoid the nasolabial fold to avoid deepening it. The sutures should drag the malar pad from above (see Fig. 2).

Complications are as mentioned previously: palpable knots, bruising, extrusion of suture ends with APTOS, and terminal dimpling. Sometimes with the stitch lift, there can be too much of a lateral vector that produces too much broadening of the face and has a tendency to flatten the malar pads.

Adjustable vector midface lift

Another suture suspension technique, described by Dr. Joe Niamtu [6,7], is particularly applicable to malar elevation. Dr. Niamtu described an intraoral approach to expose the malar fat pad, and a suture is fixed to the inferior pole. Instrumentation, passed from an access wound in the temple across the zygomatic arch and into the intraoral wound, is used to grasp the sutures, which are then brought out at the temple wound and fixed to the temporalis fascia after elevating the midface into the desired position

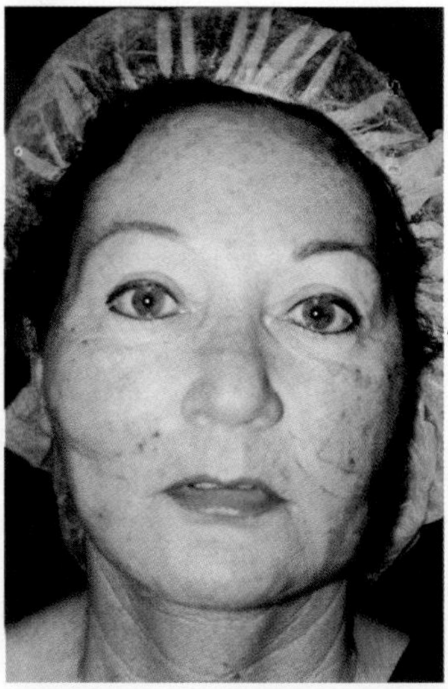

Fig. 12. Intraoperative photo showing only the right side of the face elevated with APTOS, displaying the range of lift achievable.

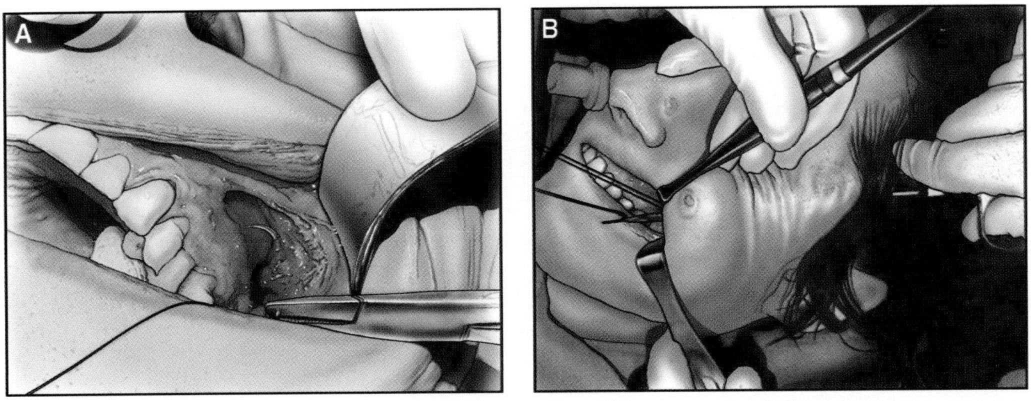

Fig. 13. (*A*, *B*) The adjustable vector midface lift. (Courtesy of J. Niamtu, DDS, Richmond, VA.)

(Fig. 13). Subtle adjustments of the vectors allow for a more vertical elevation or a slightly more superolateral repositioning.

Although this technique differs from the earlier-described lifts by virtue of the manner and degree of dissection, it is still a suture suspension lift and has the particular advantages of a deeper plane of lift with good volumetric changes to the malar pads and a secure anchor point.

Of note, in malar enhancement, clinicians should consider adding volume to the malar pad or softening the nasolabial fold using a dermal filler such as polyacrylamide gel or polylactic acid. This process invariably adds an extra element to the final appearance. Flattening of the cheeks is a classic stigma of an aging face and, without added volume, usually remains undercorrected (Fig. 14).

It is important to note that a slight bend in the spinal needle will negotiate the curve required in the Feather Lift malar placement (Fig. 15).

Jowls

The marionette lines and the fold immediately lateral to these are particularly despised by patients

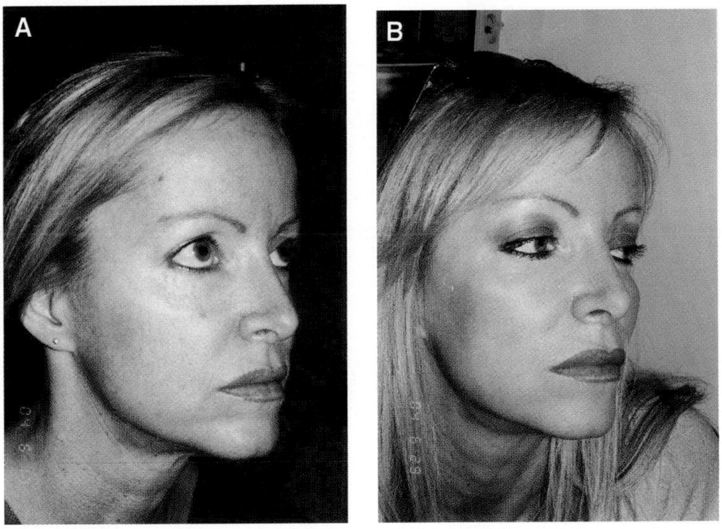

Fig. 14. Before (*A*) and after (*B*) combination of APTOS threads and malar enhancement with polyacrylamide gel.

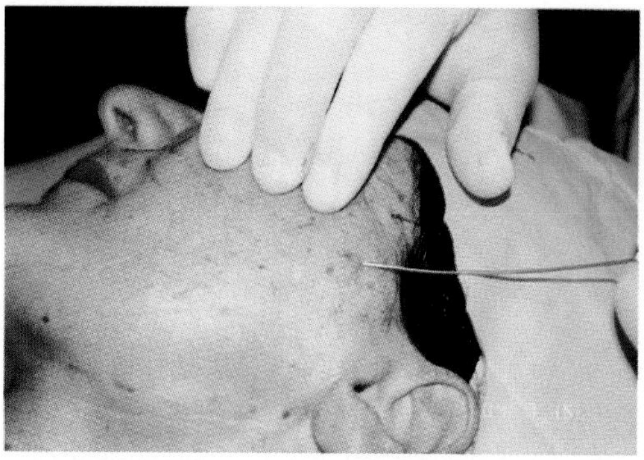

Fig. 15. A slight bend in the spinal needle often helps with the placement of threads, particularly negotiating the front curve of the malar.

and are difficult to correct. The placement of the APTOS threads described in the Feather Lift show a sharply curved course in the lower portion. This degree of curve is difficult to achieve unless the needle is introduced inferiorly and passed superiorly. The author finds that placing the introducer in a finer curve from superior to inferior allows better placement and provides a more superolateral vector. If the inferior end of the APTOS is placed too low or even beyond the marionette line, then on retraction, the prominence of this fold can be increased. The point of purchase should be lateral to the marionette fold, not in it. Alterations in the placement of APTOS compared with the Feather Lift can give a more vertical vector without the risk of pulling and thus distorting the corner of the mouth.

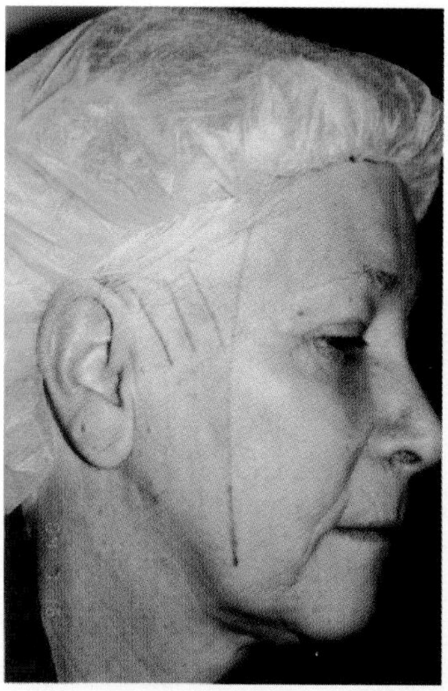

Fig. 16. In this patient, there is marked loss of preauricular hair from a face-lift procedure performed elsewhere some years previously. The markings show the placements for the loop sutures for a stitch lift tightening of the jowls. The longer thread attends directly to the jowl and the shorter threads serve to redistribute excessive laxity in the skin. Further elevation of the skin in the temple area would be inappropriate and excision of the skin would result in a visible scar, which the patient would not tolerate.

Stitch lift

In this area, the stitch lift technique is an extension of that used for the malar area but allows a more vertical vector (Fig. 16).

Neck tightening

The laxity of neck skin, particularly associated with platysma bands, is of concern to many patients.

Antiptosis suture threads

A couplet of APTOS threads threaded along the margin of the mandible and just below provides good support. The tissues are less dense here, and

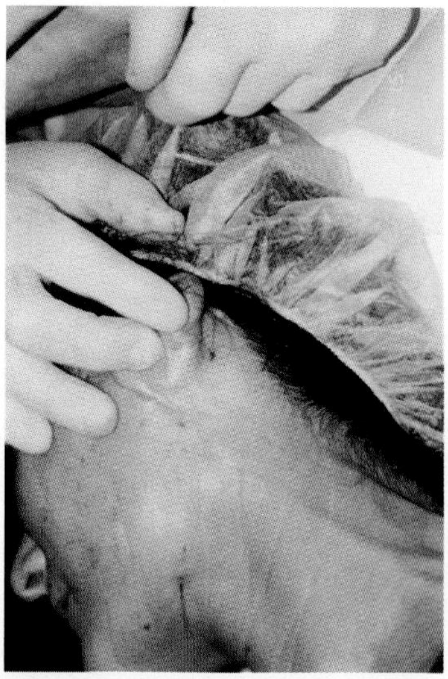

Fig. 17. Insertion of APTOS thread for neck tightening, passing below the line of the mandible and exiting in the firmer tissue over the mastoid.

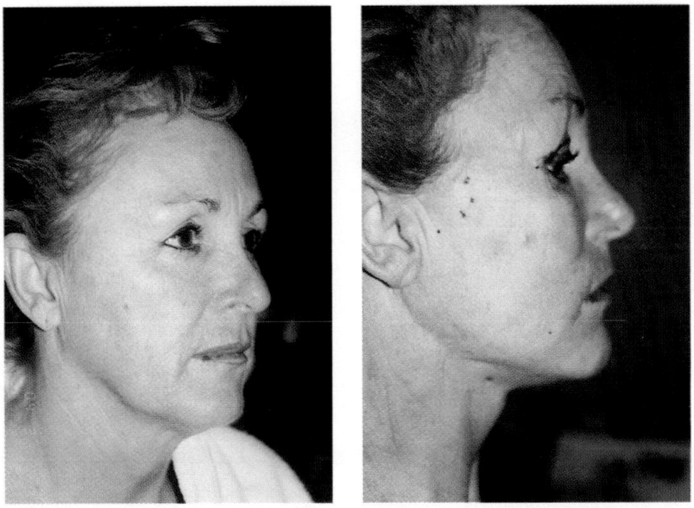

Fig. 18. Before (*left image*) and after (*right image*) APTOS threads for cheek and jowl with SAfFE approach to neck tightening. Note the minor skin folds and retraction in the skin of the neck. The extent of this appearance will resolve spontaneously over 2 to 3 weeks without intervention.

placement of the APTOS in the correct layer is important. The author finds this area to be the most difficult for obtaining persistently good results with APTOS. It appears that there is no good anchor point. The APTOS must be passed well behind the ear to lodge in the more dense tissue over the mastoid for the barbs to have any reasonable anchor (Fig. 17).

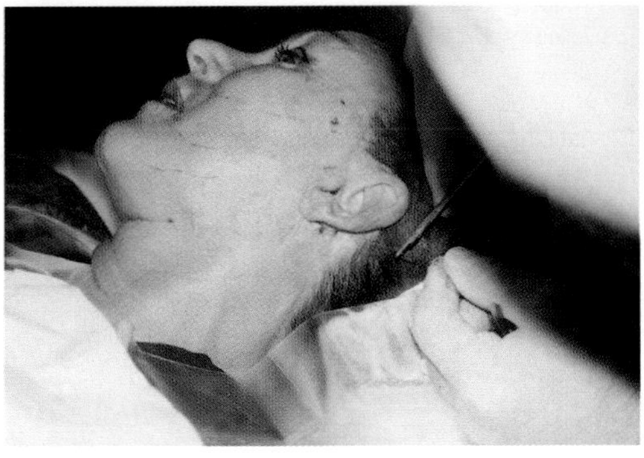

Fig. 19. Neck tightening with SAfFE approach. Note the exit of the filaments well behind the ear with the secure anchoring to the fascia over the mastoid process.

Secure anchoring filaments for facial elevation lift

The SAfFE lift technique works very well in the neck area, and the mastoid fascia provides a strong anchor point (Figs. 18 and 19).

Combination procedures

As often happens in medicine, there is rarely a single procedure that works in isolation to correct every problem. Suture suspension techniques are particularly useful in the right candidate. Their limitations are seen when used in "fringe" candidates and usually relate to problems of skin quality or lack of volume. Skin redundancy is also an issue. Skin programs to rejuvenate, such as peels, resurfacing, or nonablative rejuvenating procedures, should be considered in pertinent cases and attempted before undertaking the suture suspension because vigorous facial manipulation soon after an APTOS procedure or other technique is counterproductive. Volumetric enhancement over and above the thread techniques is helpful in achieving the desired youthful curves. Injectable facial fillers can be used before or after the "threads," although there should be an interval of several weeks after threads. Larger volume replacement (particularly in the malar area) such as autologous fat transfer is often better done before the thread procedure.

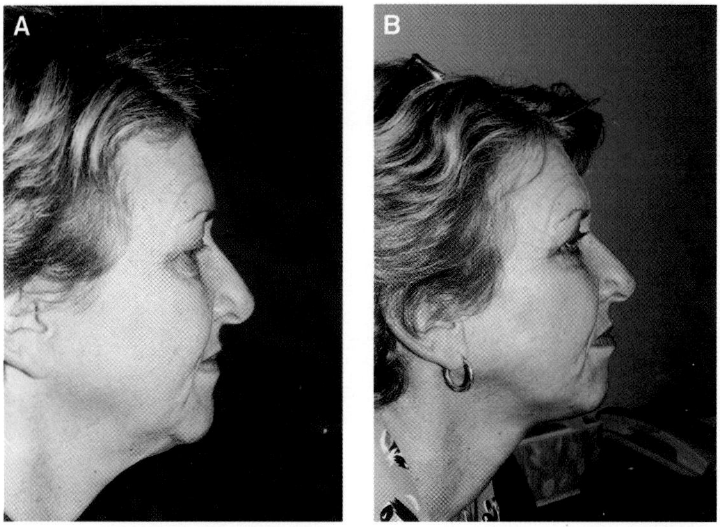

Fig. 20. Before (*A*) and after (*B*) combination of Giampappa suture and stitch lift for neck tightening. Giampappa suture improves the cervicomental angle and the stitch lift tightens the skin. A postauricular incision allows a small skin excision to avoid a roll of redundant tissue without an obvious scar.

Skin redundancy is sometimes sufficient to require excision, but the placement of a surgical scar obviates the prime advantage of undertaking the suture suspension technique in the first place. In the temple, the scar can be hidden in the hairline. In the neck, which can be a particularly difficult area when there is significant skin laxity, the scar can be placed in the postauricular sulcus and be well hidden (Fig. 20).

Summary

The author commends the various suture suspension techniques discussed, provided care is exercised in candidate selection. It is equally imperative to manage the expectations of the patient. There are some patients who expect a face-lift–type result from a suture suspension procedure, which is likely to result in disappointment. The clinician needs to portray a reasonable expectation, and in so doing, will have a better chance of a satisfied patient.

References

[1] Giampappa VC, Di Bernado BE. Neck recontouring with suture suspension and liposuction: an alternative for early rhytidectomy candidate. Aesth Plast Surg 1995; 19:217–23.
[2] Saylan Z. The S Lift: less is more. Aesth Surg J 1999; 19(5):406.
[3] Sulimanidze MA, Fournier PF, Paikidze TG, et al. Removal of facial soft tissue ptosis with special threads. Derm Surg 2002;5(28):367–71.
[4] Fragen R. Available at: www.featherlift.com.
[5] Fernandes D. Eyebrow lifting and a simple method for correction of ectropion and entropion. Proceedings of the Australasian College of Cosmetic Surgery and Cosmetic Physicians Society of Australasia Combined Annual Meeting. Gold Coast, Australia, August 2003.
[6] Niamtu J, Chisholm B. The adjustable vector deep plane midface lift. J Oral Maxillofac Surg 2004;62: 630–7.
[7] Niamtu J. A simple technique for adjustable vector midface lift. Plastic Surgery Products. Los Angeles, CA: Medical World Publications; 2004.

ELSEVIER
SAUNDERS

Oral Maxillofacial Surg Clin N Am 17 (2005) 77 – 84

ORAL AND MAXILLOFACIAL SURGERY CLINICS of North America

Facial Implants: Facial Augmentation and Volume Restoration

Bruce B. Chisholm, MD, DDS

39-300 Bob Hope Drive, Suite 1208, Rancho Mirage, CA 92270, USA

Historically, aesthetic facial surgery has been dominated by skin tightening and tissue removal procedures. The face-lift procedure was first described as the elevation, tightening, and excision of skin. Over the following decades, this procedure changed considerably. The procedure now includes tightening of skin and deep structures, excision of excess tissue, composite or multiplane dissection, repositioning of ptotic tissue, and restoration of volume [1,2]. Tension restoration surgery continues to be useful but is most effective when combined with volume restoration [3–6].

Aging changes in the facial region are only partially caused by laxity of the skin and subcutaneous tissue. Loss of volume and volume shift occur in all regions of the face and neck and contribute significantly to the aged appearance [5,6] (Fig. 1). Multiple changes occur on the cellular and macroscopic levels. The soft tissue undergoes change throughout the patient's life, with acceleration in the 30s and dramatic escalation in the 40s and subsequent decades.

The changes that occur in the skin and in the deeper soft tissue structures are a consequence of the patient's genetics and lifestyle. The soft tissue envelope that encircles the bony skeleton slowly collapses. The loss of volume and the diminished support of the soft tissue result in accentuation of the aging process, with the deepening of rhytids and the inferior migration of the soft tissue. These same changes occur throughout the patient's body. The full fibrous tissue associated with youthful appearance is replaced by a less dense, less supple, and less supported tissue.

The aging upper eyelid is characterized by excess skin and soft tissue, diminishing soft tissue support, and a ptotic brow that is commonly addressed surgically by a traditional excisional blepharoplasty and endoscopic brow-lift. In addition to the excess soft tissue, there is a substantial loss of volume in the periorbital and brow region. The volume loss results in less support for the brow tissue and eyelid, with the resulting appearance of an aged periocular region (Fig. 2). Rhytids are accentuated. The ideal treatment for this region is to conservatively remove the excess skin and soft tissue, reposition or conservatively remove postseptal fat, resupport the region through volume restoration, resupport the brow with a brow-lift, and rejuvenate the skin. Autologous fat is a choice for volume restoration. Several augmentations with fat are necessary, and long-term outcomes are variable. Irregularities are not uncommon.

Aging of the lower eyelids occurs secondary to the downward and inward migration of tissue, pseudoherniation of fat, diminished soft tissue support, and actinic damage. Ideally, the treatment of the lower eyelid is resuspension of tissue (including the skin, muscle, and associated structures), repositioning or conservative excision of the postseptal fat, restoration of volume, and rejuvenation of the skin. Restoration of volume can be difficult. The loss of volume occurs at multiple levels, and current technology does not allow the problem to be effectively addressed in a fully predictable manner. The medial tear trough remains the most recalcitrant. Autologous augmentation is accomplished with fat, dermis, fascia, muscle, or a combination of these tissues.

E-mail address: bchish9127@aol.com

1042-3699/05/$ – see front matter
doi:10.1016/j.coms.2004.10.004

oralmaxsurgery.theclinics.com

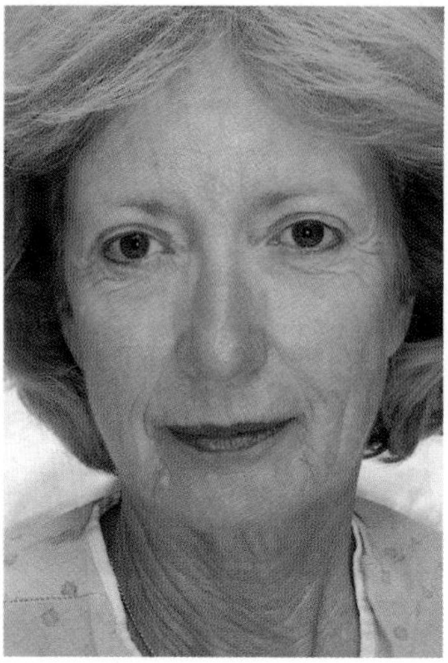

Fig. 1. Photograph illustrating loss of volume with volume shift in the face and neck region.

Restoration of the suborbital region is accomplished by suspension of tissue in the suborbital region and midface. Surgical procedures lead to partial restoration of volume. The most common method used for additional volume enhancement is conservative autologous fat augmentation; however, the problems with fat augmentation include the need for multiple procedures, the high reabsorption rate, irregularities, and patient dissatisfaction. Currently, autologous fat or soft tissue augmentation is the most frequently used method for volume restoration in the upper and lower eyelids and the periorbital region. Additional materials for augmentation include other autologous tissue; alloplastic materials such as hyaluronic acid, hydroxylapatite, or collagen; and alloplastic periorbital implants such as the tear trough implant.

Volume restoration is an important adjunct to rejuvenation of the periorbital area. Problems persist with the quality and longevity of the implant materials used and the patient's acceptance of multiple procedures or irregularities in this area. Volume restoration, in addition to the resuspension and removal of excess tissue, remains the current goal of aesthetic surgery and, in the future, will play an even greater role as implant materials improve and the science of tissue engineering advances.

The midface, malar, and submalar region is an area that is well suited to alloplastic augmentation [7]. Aging that occurs in the midface has been treated using various surgical techniques. Procedures include the temporal and lower eyelid approaches to a midface lift and suspension of subcutaneous tissue by way of a face-lift procedure. Examination of the midface region reveals that excessive tissue is rarely the most significant problem in this region. Aging in this region is greatly due to soft tissue atrophy, loss of volume, and soft tissue ptosis, particularly in the submalar region. Surgery techniques will often not adequately restore volume to this area. Additional restoration of the volume is best achieved with an alloplastic implant. Autologous implants such as fat also are effective for restoration, although they do not last as long and are not as predictable.

Patients 40 years and older often seek treatment for aging in the midface region. Those patients who have adequate malar projection are treated with submalar implants. The submalar implant is best described as an implant that restores the volume the patient has lost with age. This method is in contrast to alloplastic malar augmentation, which generally changes a patient's appearance while augmenting volume. Volume is lost in the malar region but is significantly less than the volume lost in the submalar region (see Fig. 2). The submalar implant is placed through an intraoral approach using a small incision. The implant is placed in an exact subperiosteal pocket. The amount of volume replacement that is achieved depends on the type and size of implant used. Smaller implants generally restore a former

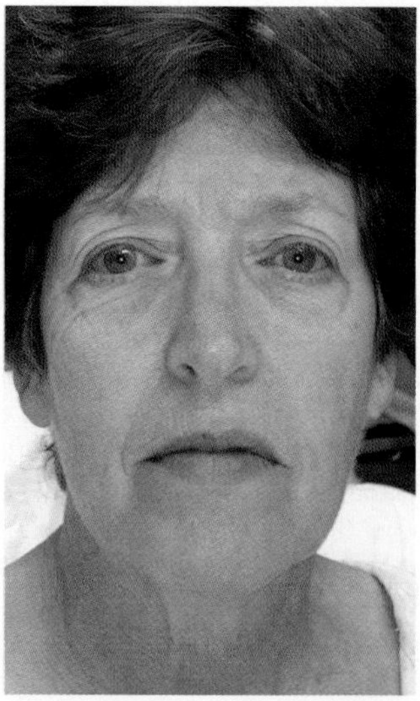

Fig. 2. Photograph showing the loss of volume in the brow and preauricular region.

appearance, whereas larger implants change an appearance and restore volume.

The area of maximum midface atrophy in most patients is in the submalar zone. The maximum projection of the submalar implant is placed immediately behind this region in a subperiosteal pocket. The implant tail is placed over the inferior edge of the zygomatic arch above the attachment of the masseter muscle. If an exact subperiosteal pocket is developed, then no fixation other than sutures is required. If a large dissection is required for placement, however, then screw fixation should be used. Restoration of volume in this area enhances the patient's postoperative appearance, adds to the cosmetic outcome of the face-lift, and enhances the longevity of the procedure. The importance of the rounded, smooth submalar zone is clearly appreciated in the youthful face. In this region, restoration of volume is often more important than a tissue tightening or removal procedure. Augmentation of the midface may also be accomplished with implants other than submalar implants. The shell implant or the malar implant may also be used. The preoperative evaluation of the patient distinguishes the areas that are atrophic or the region for which the patient is requesting augmentation.

During the aging process, the submalar region is the area where the most volume and fullness is lost or changed. The most common implant for restoration of a patient's previous appearance in this region is the submalar implant. The amount of augmentation that is used is the surgeon's and the patient's choice. Implants range from small to large. Most female patients are treated with a small submalar implant. The medium implant is most frequently used in the male patient. The sizes and shapes of the implants vary according to the manufacturer. If the patient is looking for replacement of atrophic losses that occur with aging, the smaller implant is preferable. A larger implant is reserved for the patient who desires to not only replace volume that has been lost but also augment an appearance that was previously unsatisfactory to the patient. Congenital deformities may also require a larger implant.

The traditional face-lift procedure is a tension or excisional procedure. Volume restoration is as important as the tension/excisional procedure. The loss of volume accentuates the downward and inward migration of soft tissue, provides less support for overlying skin, and expedites the onset and deepening of rhytids. Rhytids are a function of muscle contraction and folding of the skin but they are deepened and their formation is accelerated by the loss of volume.

Aging changes that occur in the perioral region are multifactorial and complex. Deep rhytids, loss of volume, and laxity of the tissue contribute to the appearance of aging in this region. The traditional tightening or tension procedures are less important than restoration of volume and treatment of damaged skin. Rhytids in this area are primarily due to the function of the perioral muscles, particularly the orbicularis oris. Actinically damaged skin and loss of volume also are significant. Many surgeons have been frustrated in their attempts to treat the perioral region when volume restoration is not considered. Restoring volume is the single most important factor when treating the nasolabial regions, marionette lines, and the downward sloping corners of the mouth. Volume restoration may be achieved with autologous fat, hydroxylapatite, hyaluronic acid, collagen, autologous dermal and fascial tissue, or other fillers. An effective treatment of the area is traditional face-lifting to tighten and remove excess skin, perioral augmentation of volume with autologous fat or hydroxylapatite, midface augmentation with an alloplastic implant, skin resurfacing, and individual rhytid treatment with hydroxylapatite.

Microgenia is effectively addressed with alloplastic augmentation [8,9]. The other option is an osteotomy. The osteotomy has a higher complication rate, moves an abnormal structure forward, and may be more difficult to perform for many surgeons. Notching and irregularities are common. The placement of an extended alloplastic anatomic chin implant is a simple, safe, and easily performed procedure.The implant is placed through a small skin incision in the submental region [10]. An exact periosteal

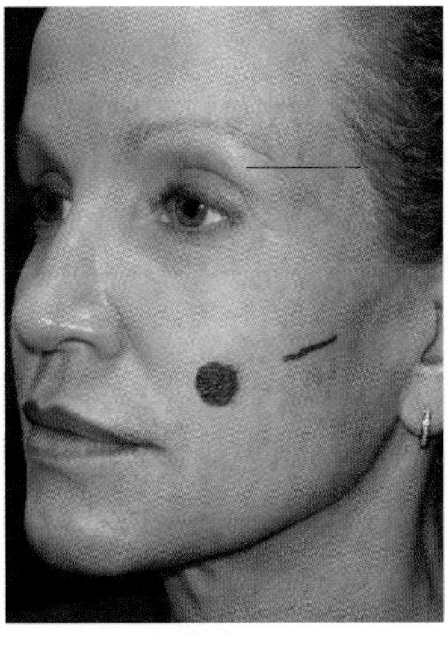

Fig. 3. Preoperative markings of the atrophic submalar region and zygomatic arch.

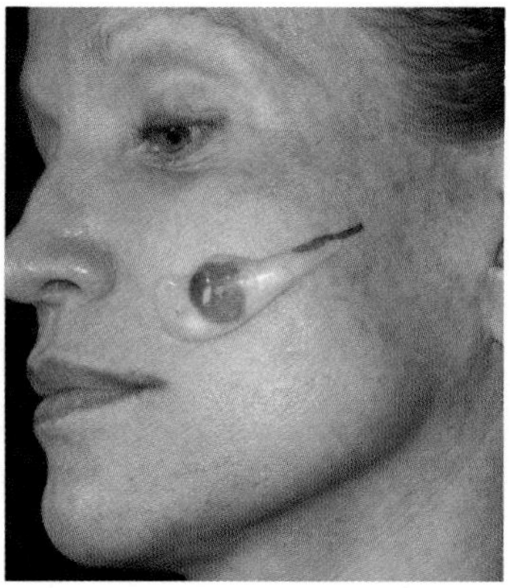

Fig. 4. Silastic submalar implant placed over the submalar region.

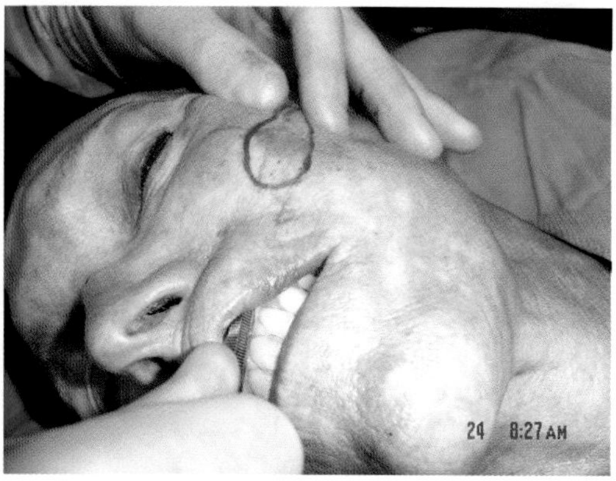

Fig. 6. The subperiosteal implant pocket developed with a periosteal elevator.

pocket is developed and the implant is placed and secured. The patient's appearance is greatly enhanced by restoring the chin and cervicomental region [11,12].

Implant materials for chin augmentation include Silicone, GORE-TEX, and porous polyethylene. Porous materials will make removal or revision of the implants difficult [8]. Bone resorption is a result of pressure and muscle function. In a patient with a severely deficient chin and a hypertrophic mentalis muscle, there may be resorption of underlying bone. Most patients with a mild to moderately deficient chin are well treated with an alloplastic implant [8]. Postoperatively, if a nonporous material becomes a problem, it is easily repositioned or removed.

Aging also leads to loss of volume in the soft tissue chin region. The ptosis and loss of soft tissue support can be improved with volume restoration. If the patient has microgenia, then a chin implant combined with soft tissue filling and tension restoration is most effective.

Procedure

Submalar

With the patient in the sitting position, the atrophic submalar area is marked (Fig. 3) and the

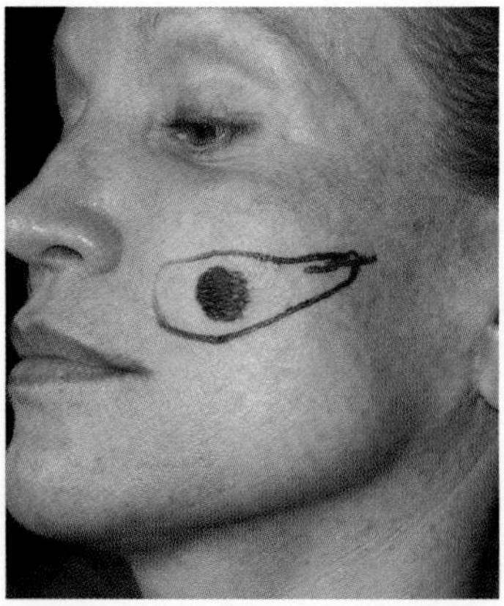

Fig. 5. Outline drawn on the skin for submalar implant placement.

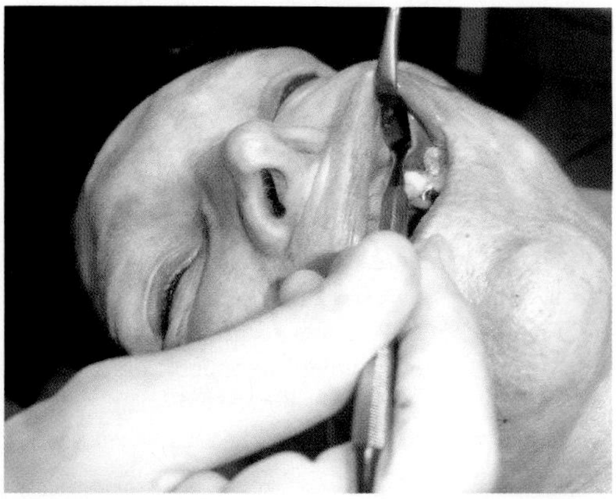

Fig. 7. Placement of submalar implant using right-angled retractor.

zygomatic arch is outlined. After establishing appropriate anesthesia and assuring surgical sterility and technique, the implant is placed on the patient's cheek. The implant is placed with its maximum projection over the previously marked atrophic region (Fig. 4) and outlined using a marking pen (Fig. 5). Intraorally, a small incision is made with Iris scissors in the canine fossa. A No. 9 periosteal elevator is used to elevate an exact periosteal pocket following the outline drawn on the patient's skin (Fig. 6). The implant is kept soaking in antibiotic solution. Using a small right-angled retractor, the implant is placed under direct vision (Fig. 7). After the position is assured, the implant is secured with a reabsorbable suture. When the implant pocket has been enlarged more than a few millimeters beyond the implant, the implant should be secured with screws. The wound is closed with reabsorbable sutures in two layers. It is important to place the incision anteriorly and make it small in size to ensure that the implant does not sit

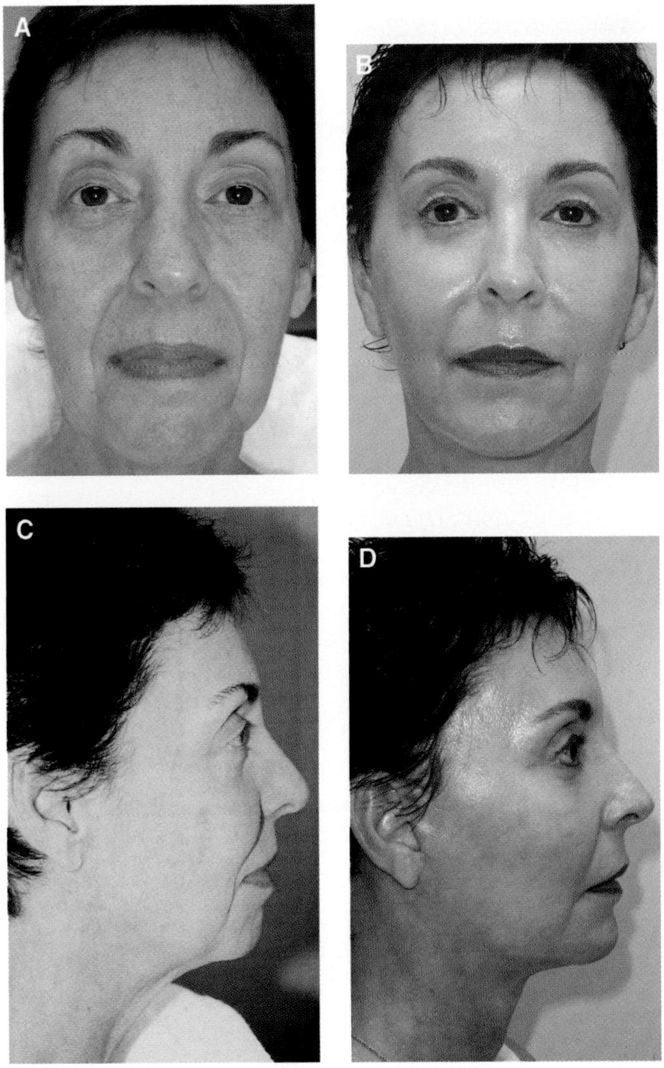

Fig. 8. Preoperative frontal (*A*) and lateral (*C*) view. Six-months postoperative frontal (*B*) and lateral (*D*) view following facelift, Endo brow-lift, upper-eyelid blepharoplasty, submalar implants, Silastic chin implant, skin resurfacing, and rhinoplasty.

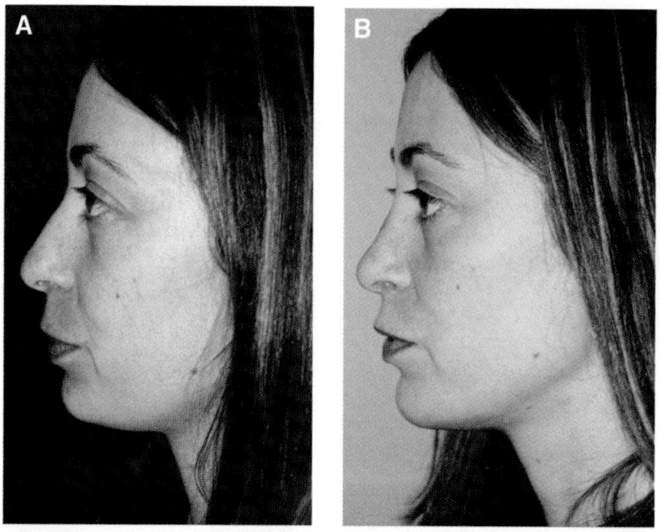

Fig. 9. (*A*) Preoperative view. (*B*) One-year postoperative view following Silastic anatomic chin implant and rhinoplasty.

on the incision and cause breakdown, dehiscence, and infection.

Chin

After adequate anesthesia is established and sterile technique is assured, a small incision is made in the submental crease. Under direct vision, the periosteum is elevated. The inferior of the anterior border of the mandible is dissected in the subperiosteal plane with a No. 9 periosteal elevator. Dissection is continued along the lateral borders with external finger control of the instrument at all times to avoid mental nerve injury. Anteriorly, the dissection is widened to

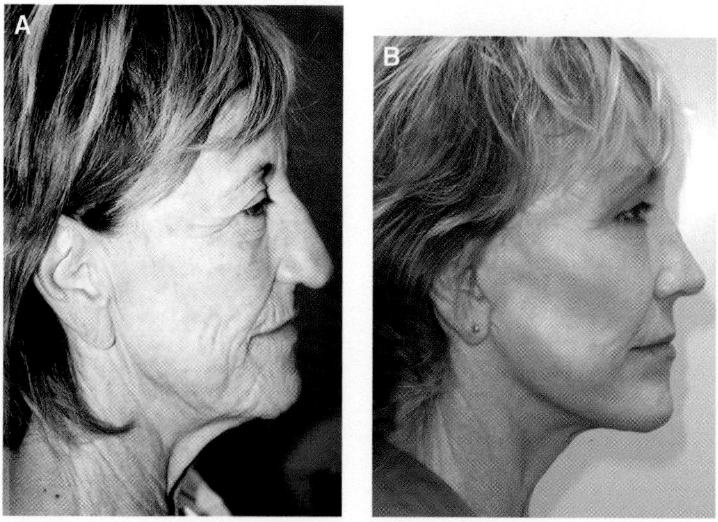

Fig. 10. (*A*) Preoperative view. (*B*) Ten-months postoperative view following face-lift, Endo brow-lift, upper-eyelid blepharoplasty, submalar implants, and skin resurfacing, and rhinoplasty.

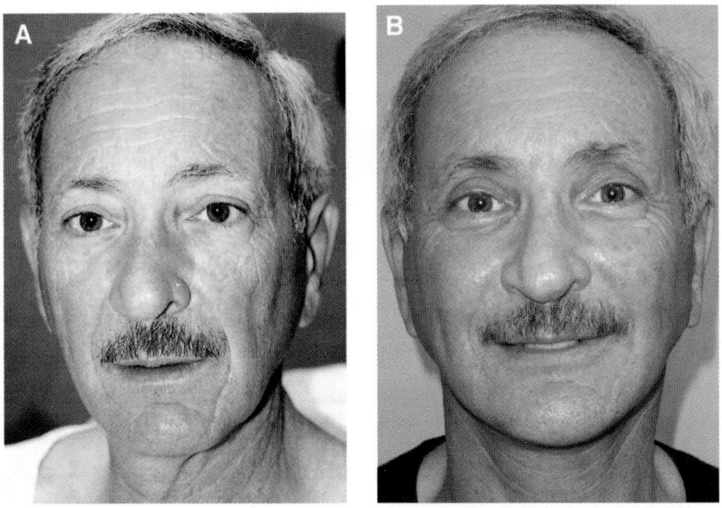

Fig. 11. (*A*) Preoperative view. (*B*) Eight-months postoperative view following face-lift, upper-eyelid blepharoplasty, submalar implants, and skin resurfacing.

accommodate the body of the implant. The tips of the anatomic Silicone implants [8,13] are conservatively trimmed because they are thin and may protrude into the soft tissue. The implant is placed in the pocket using a small right-angled retractor. Four 5-0 reabsorbable sutures are used to secure the implant. Screws may also be used. The incision is closed in layers with 6-0 reabsorbable suture in the deep layers and 6-0 nonabsorbable suture on the skin.

Summary

The addition of volume restoration has advanced facial aesthetic surgery. Tightening and removal of excess skin and resuspension of deep tissues such as the malar fat and muscles are important in restoration of the face. Improved aesthetic outcomes occur, however, when volume restoration is also achieved (Figs. 8–11). The longevity of the surgical procedure is enhanced with volume restoration. Complications are minimal (Table 1).

Table 1
Complications with chin and submalar implants

Complication	Silastic chin (n = 95)	Silastic submalar (n = 415)
Infection	0	0
Implant loss	0	0
Permanent dysesthesia	0	0
Implant malposition (requiring reposition)	1	0

References

[1] Hamra ST. The zygorbicular dissection in composite rhytidectomy: an ideal midface plane. Plast Reconstr Surg 1998;102(5):1646–57.
[2] Ramirez OM. The subperiosteal rhytidectomy: the third generation facelift. Ann Plast Surg 1992;28:218.
[3] Terino EO. The art of alloplastic facial contouring. St. Louis (MO): Mosby; 2000.
[4] Terino EO. Facial contouring with alloplastic implants: aesthetic surgery that creates three dimensions. Facial Plast Surg 1999;7:55–83.
[5] Constantinides MS, Doud-Galli SK, Miller PJ, et al. Malar, submalar, midfacial implants. Facial Plast Surg 2000;16:35–44.
[6] Terino EO. Alloplastic facial contouring by zonal principles of skeletal anatomy. Clin Plast Surg 1992; 19:487.
[7] Metzinger SE, McCollough G, Campbell JP, et al. Malar augmentation: a 5 year retrospective review of the Silastic midfacial malar implant. Arch Otolaryngol Head Neck Surg 1998;125:980–7.
[8] Zide BM, Pfeifer TM, Longaker MT. Chin surgery: I. Augmentation—the allures and the alerts. Plast Reconstr Surg 1999;104:1843.

[9] Tardy ME, Thomas JR, Brown RJ. Facial aesthetic surgery. St. Louis (MO): Mosby; 1995.
[10] Zide BM. The mentalis muscle: an essential component of chin and lower lip position. Plast Reconstr Surg 2000;105:1213.
[11] Auger TA, Turley PK. The female soft tissue profile as presented in fashion magazines during the 1900's. A photographic analysis. Intern J Adult Orthodon Orthognath Surg 1999;14:7–18.
[12] Perrett DI, May KA, Yoshodawa S. Facial shape and judgements of female attractiveness. Nature 1994;368: 239–42.
[13] Vuyk HD. Augmentation mentoplasty with solid silicone. Clin Otolaryngol 1996;21:106–18.

ELSEVIER
SAUNDERS

Oral Maxillofacial Surg Clin N Am 17 (2005) 85 – 98

ORAL AND
MAXILLOFACIAL
SURGERY CLINICS
of North America

Submentoplasty and Facial Liposuction

L. Angelo Cuzalina, MD, DDS[a,b,c,*], James Koehler, MD, DDS[a,c]

[a]*Tulsa Surgical Arts, 7316 East 91st Street, Tulsa, OK 74133, USA*
[b]*Department of Oral and Maxillofacial Surgery, University of Oklahoma, 1201 North Stonewall Avenue, P.O. Box 26901, Oklahoma City, OK 73190, USA*
[c]*Department of Oral and Maxillofacial Surgery, University of Alabama, SDB419, 1919 7th Avenue South, Birmingham, AL 35235, USA*

The demand for esthetic procedures has increased with the increased public awareness of the results that can be achieved. Patients frequently request a more defined jaw line, removal of excess submental fat, and improvement in submental skin laxity. A variety of procedures are available; however, it is important to properly diagnose the patient and select the appropriate procedure to obtain maximal results.

Patients who complain of poor neck contour are often shocked when a face-lift is the procedure recommended by the surgeon. Often, the patient is not prepared to undergo a more invasive procedure but still desires improvement in neck contour.

The goal of this article is to provide the surgeon with information on appropriate patient selection and current techniques for less invasive procedures such as liposuction or submentoplasty to improve aesthetics of certain neck conditions. It is important for the surgeon to recognize the limitations of these procedures and counsel patients appropriately.

Patient assessment

The initial workup involves taking an accurate history and performing a detailed physical examination. It is important to rule out any pathologic process that can be contributing to the patient's chief complaint of submental fullness and poor neck contour, such as thyroid hyperplasia or salivary gland pathology. After ensuring that no pathology is present, it is important to evaluate the cosmetic imperfections (Fig. 1) [1].

First, the surgeon should look at the patient's skin tone and laxity. In general, a younger patient with good skin tone is a better candidate for liposuction. If the patient has tremendous skin laxity, then less dramatic improvement can be achieved with liposuction even when a significant amount of submental fat is present. The surgeon can determine the amount of preplatysmal fat by gently pinching the skin with his or her fingers. If there is still sufficient fullness with this maneuver, then the patient may also have significant deposits of subplatysmal fat that cannot properly be addressed with liposuction alone and a submentoplasty should be considered.

Next, the position of the hyoid bone should be noted by palpation. A low- and anterior-positioned hyoid bone results in an obtuse cervicomental angle despite good surgical techniques to treat the submental region (Fig. 2). Recognizing this preoperatively allows the surgeon to discuss the limitations of the procedure or alternatives such as camouflaging with a chin implant [2].

Signs of an aging neck include jowling and platysmal banding (see Fig. 1). Jowling appears as fullness in the posterior mandibular region from loss of muscle tone and skin elasticity. Platysmal banding occurs as a result of a weakened platysmal muscle

* Corresponding author. American Academy Cosmetic Surgery Fellowship, Tulsa Surgical Arts, 7316 East 91st Street, Tulsa, OK 74133.

E-mail address: angelo@tulsasurgicalarts.com (L.A. Cuzalina).

1042-3699/05/$ – see front matter
doi:10.1016/j.coms.2004.09.008

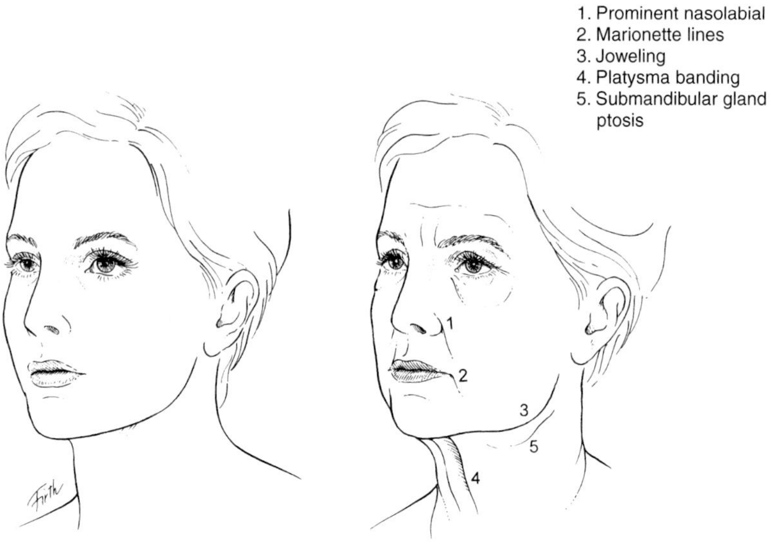

Fig. 1. Typical features of aging in the lower facial third and neck.

and dehiscence of the fibers in the midline of the neck. Although platysmal banding can dramatically be improved with an aggressive submentoplasty, it must be remembered that the most appropriate procedure for combined jowling and platysmal banding or laxity often is a cervicofacial rhytidectomy with or without a concurrent submentoplasty.

It is also important to recognize submandibular gland ptosis; that is, when the submandibular gland is visible as a small chestnut-sized mass in the neck several centimeters below the angle of the mandible (see Fig. 1). If gland ptosis is unrecognized, then the esthetic result will be less than satisfactory with traditional liposuction and submentoplasty. In fact, aggressive liposuction may cause the patient to recognize submandibular gland ptosis that they did not notice preoperatively. Traditionally, the patient is informed of the limitations or an attempt is made at suspension of the gland [3]. Currently, the authors manage this problem with partial submandibular gland resection through a submental crease. This technique is discussed later in this article. If the ptotic

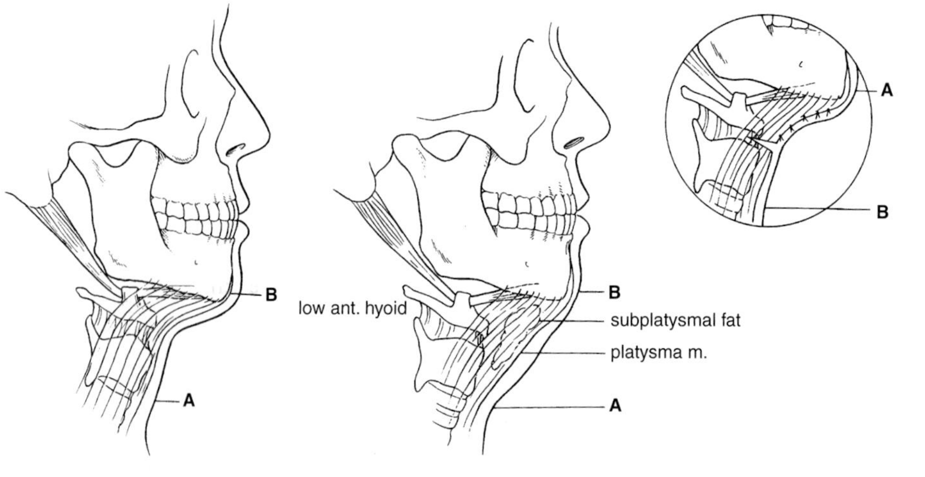

Fig. 2. (*Left*) Normal hyoid position and cervicomental angle. (*Center*) Low and anterior hyoid position with obtuse cervicomental angle. (*Right*) After submentoplasty including platysmaplasty and plication. Note that the length from A to B is the same; therefore, no skin resection is required to obtain an improved cervicomental angle. Adequate amounts of pre- and subplatysmal fat must be resected for the skin to properly redrape. ant., anterior; m., muscle.

gland is not addressed, then the patient will have a residual bulge in the submandibular triangle that may be more noticeable after excessive fat has been reduced by surgery.

Liposuction

After systematic patient evaluation, the decision needs to be made regarding whether the patient's neck can be treated with liposuction alone, liposuction with submentoplasty, or submentoplasty with traditional rhytidectomy. The ideal candidate for liposuction is usually a patient less than 40 years old who has good skin tone, a favorable hyoid position, and localized submental and submandibular fat deposits [4]. When there is minor platysmal banding, consideration for botulinum toxin type A (Botox) injections to the platysma with liposuction can be considered [5]; however, significant platysmal banding or laxity will need to be treated with submentoplasty.

The technique for cervicofacial liposuction has evolved over the years [6–15]. Previously, surgeons used large spatulated cannulas to extract as much fat as possible from the neck. The initial results were often good, but over time, patients developed a skeletonized appearance of the neck. Also, it is very easy to create an uneven removal of fat and develop a lumpy appearance. Today, the trend is to use small cannulas 1 to 2 mm in diameter. The goal for cervicofacial liposuction is to resculpt the neck to improve the contour, not to remove all the fat [16].

Preoperatively, patients are informed that after fat is removed by liposuction, it is expected that the skin will shrink to take on the new contour. It is important to warn the patient that if excess skin laxity develops after the procedure, then additional surgical procedures may be required.

Tumescent solution

Tumescent anesthesia was first described in the dermatology literature as a technique in which liposuction could be performed safely under local anesthesia alone. It was found that using a dilute solution of lidocaine and epinephrine decreased the blood loss during liposuction and provided safety to the technique [17–19]. Even though there is minimal blood loss with submental liposuction, tumescent anesthesia distends the tissue plane between the platysma and the skin and facilitates the liposuction procedure [20].

Facial liposuction is considered small-volume liposuction because the amount removed is typically less than 100 mL. Liposuction is considered large volume when 1500 to 4000 mL supernatant fat is removed in one session. Removing more than 4 L in one session is reported to have increased risk of complications such as fluid shifts, deep venous thrombosis, and pulmonary embolism. The risks involved with facial liposuction are extremely low.

One of the principle drugs in the tumescent solution is lidocaine. In the *Physicians' Desk Reference*, the maximum safe dose of lidocaine is 7 mg/kg. This dose limit was established in 1948 by a letter to the Food and Drug Administration from Astra Pharmaceuticals that stated the safe dose of lidocaine was "probably the same as that for procainamide" [21]. Dr. Klein challenged this dogma and developed the tumescent anesthesia technique for liposuction in 1986.

Through well-documented prospective studies, an estimated safe upper dose of lidocaine, in highly dilute form, used for body liposuction has been validated at 35 mg/kg [22]. This dose is five times the limit published previously. For body liposuction, the current estimate for the safe maximum dose of lidocaine is 50 mg/kg; doses greater than 55 mg/kg should be avoided [21,23,24]. In 20 patients, when doses of lidocaine in the range of 50 mg/kg were administered, peak serum blood levels were noted to be less than 3.5 μg/mL. The toxic serum threshold is reported to be 5 μg/mL. It is important to note that peak lidocaine levels do not occur until 12 hours after administration during tumescent technique for body liposuction [25].

The situation is slightly different in the face. Much lower amounts of solution are injected in the face, and the dose of lidocaine should never approach the levels used in body liposuction. Due to its excellent blood supply, it is not surprising that the face has a much faster rate of absorption. Serial plasma lidocaine levels have been measured when using tumescent anesthesia on the face. In one study, the peak plasma levels averaged 2.7 μg/mL, and the highest level found in the series was 3.3 μg/mL. In addition, the serum levels normally peaked at 1 hour after administration rather than 12 hours with body tumescence [26].

Epinephrine is essential to the mixture of tumescent anesthesia. It provides the profound vasoconstriction mediated by alpha-1 agonist effects that limits blood loss during liposuction. In addition, epinephrine decreases the rate of absorption of lidocaine, thereby decreasing systemic toxicity [27]. The most common adverse reaction to epinephrine is a tachyarrythmia related to the beta-1 agonist effects. Use of clonidine as a premedicant has been shown to greatly reduce the incidence of intraoperative and postoperative tachycardia with tumescent local.

Bicarbonate is usually added to the tumescent mixture (to reduce the stinging pain due to the acidity of lidocaine) injected in an awake patient. It is usually added to obtain a concentration of 10 mEq/L. The authors do not use bicarbonate because they perform liposuction under sedation or general anesthesia.

It should be recognized by surgeons that the original tumescent technique is done without any sedation. When sedation or general anesthesia is used, close attention to vitals and signs of toxicity should monitored [28]. In isolated facial liposuction, toxicity is unlikely to be a problem because lidocaine concentrations should be extremely low [29].

Drug interactions with tumescent

The surgeon should recognize that there are potential drug interactions [30]. Drugs that inhibit the hepatic enzymes cytochrome P-450 1A2 and 3A4 can increase lidocaine toxicity. The most common drugs that interact are the selective serotonin reuptake inhibitors (eg, Zoloft), benzodiazepines, H-2 blockers, proton pump inhibitors, antifungal medications, calcium channel blockers, and macrolide antibiotics. It has been recommended that maximum doses of lidocaine should be decreased by half for patients on drugs that inhibit cytochrome P-450 1A2 and 3A4. Because epinephrine is also used, the potential for adverse reactions is present with monoamine oxidase inbibitors, cocaine use, β-blockers, and hyperthyroidism. Appropriate caution should be used with patients on these medications. For the small doses of tumescent anesthesia administered for facial liposuction, the risk of toxicity is low, even with patients on these medications.

Technique

The patient is first marked with a permanent marker in an upright position. The areas requiring the greatest amount of liposuction are circled. Straight lines mark areas that are to be blended in a fanned pattern. Marking is important because it may be difficult to locate the areas that require the most liposuction after the patient has been insufflated with tumescent solution and placed in a supine position.

Next, the patient is sedated or placed under general anesthesia. After complete skin preparation, the submental region is infiltrated with tumescent anesthesia. The authors typically mix 30 mL 2% lidocaine (600 mg) with 1.5 mL 1:1000 epinephrine (1.5 mg) into 500 mL normal saline. This mixture makes 0.12% lidocaine with 1:333,333 epinephrine. The mixture is injected with a Wells Johnson Klein pump (Tuscon, Arizona) and a 22-gauge spinal needle into the submental region and from an area just below the pinna of the ear bilaterally. The injection is placed just superficial to the superficial musculoaponeurotic system (SMAS) in the upper face and just superficial to the platysma in the neck. Injection at deeper levels may injure nerves or vascular structures. If the injection is done too superficially, a peau d'orange appearance of the skin may be noted. This appearance should be avoided. There are reports of skin slough in face-lifting that are attributed to superficial injection of tumescent solution in areas of skin undermining. The authors have not seen this occur; however, it is important to inject the solution to the proper depth. Approximately 150 mL of tumescent solution is used in the submental region.

The skin is then reprepped and the patient is draped for the procedure. It is best to wait approximately 15 to 20 minutes after injecting the solution before beginning liposuction. Stab incisions are first made with a No. 11 scalpel blade in the submental region and just below the pinna of the ear bilaterally. For liposuction in the midfacial region, some surgeons prefer to make a stab incision just above the helix of the ear.

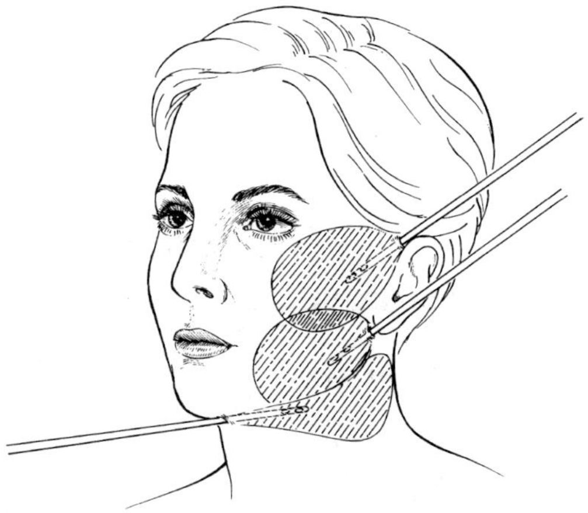

Fig. 3. Liposuction of the cheek is performed through a supra-auricular incision, liposuction of the jowls is best performed through an incision at the base of the ear lobe, and submental liposuction is best performed through a submental crease incision. Do not attempt to liposuction the jowls through a submental incision.

A small, 1.5- or 2-mm microliposuction cannula is used to perform the liposuction (Fig. 3). Small cannulas decrease the likelihood of having uneven or lumpy results. It is important that the cannula opening always be pointed toward the platysma. If the cannula is facing the skin, it can result in gouging of the dermal tissues and cause increased scarring, induration, and palpable skin irregularities. Although ultrasonic liposuction cannulas are available for facial liposuctions, their use is not indicated in this region because the amount of fat is minimal and the risk of thermal injury to dermal tissues is too great.

The cannula should be moved in a smooth in-and-out motion. Each time the cannula is pushed in; it should enter a new location. When the cannula is kept in the same area for multiple passes, irregularities develop that can be difficult to correct. The dominant hand holds the cannula and the nondominant hand should always be held gently over the skin to feel the depth of the cannula tip. In addition, the surgeon should frequently stop to feel the skin to ensure even removal of fat. The cannula tip should always be superficial to the platysma. When removal of sub-playtsmal fat is indicated, it should be done surgically because excessive bleeding and nerve injury can result if this is performed blindly.

When performing submental liposuction, it is important to not bring the liposuction cannula above the inferior border of the mandible from the submental incision. Doing so can place the facial nerve at risk. It is better to access the jowls with the liposuction cannula from the incisions below the pinna of the ear (see Fig. 3). Overly aggressive liposuction of the jowl region can result in facial nerve weakness. As mentioned before, when the cannula is not kept superficial to the platysma, facial nerve or vessel injury can occur.

After liposuction is completed, a single 5-0 plain gut suture is used to close the stab incisions. Reston foam 1563L (3M Medical-Surgical, St. Paul, Minnesota) is placed over the submental region and Coban (3M Medical-Surgical) head wrap is gently applied. This wrap is kept on for 24 hours. When the patient returns the next day, the wrap is removed and a face-lift bra is placed. This face-lift bra is to be worn as much as possible, day and night, during the first week. After 1 week, the patient is to wear the garment only at night for 2 more weeks (Figs. 4–6).

Complications reported with facial liposuction include dermal injury with postoperative indurations, skin irregularities, prolonged swelling, seromas, hematomas, sialoceles, transient and permanent injury of the marginal mandibular nerve, and post-inflammatory hyperpigmentation [31]. Induration can be improved with massage or external ultrasound therapy. Persistent localized areas of induration may improve with judicious use of injectable steroids such as small doses (0.2–0.4 mL) of triamcinolone (Kenalog), 10 mg/mL, in isolated areas of thickness. Hematomas and seromas are usually treated with serial aspiration and compression dressings; however, large hematomas may require surgical evacuation and, rarely, drain placement. Prompt attention along with frequent and thorough follow-up visits is mandatory to avoid long-term fibrotic sequelae that can be very difficult to treat. Sialoceles should not occur with proper technique; however, when a sialocele develops, the use of serial aspiration and the use of medication to decrease saliva production, such as scopolamine patches, may be helpful. Motor

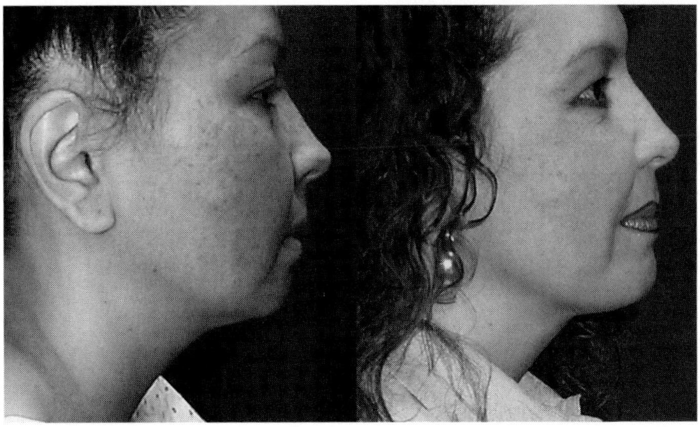

Fig. 4. Before (*left image*) and 6 months after (*right image*) isolated neck liposuction and chin implant placement on a 39-year-old woman.

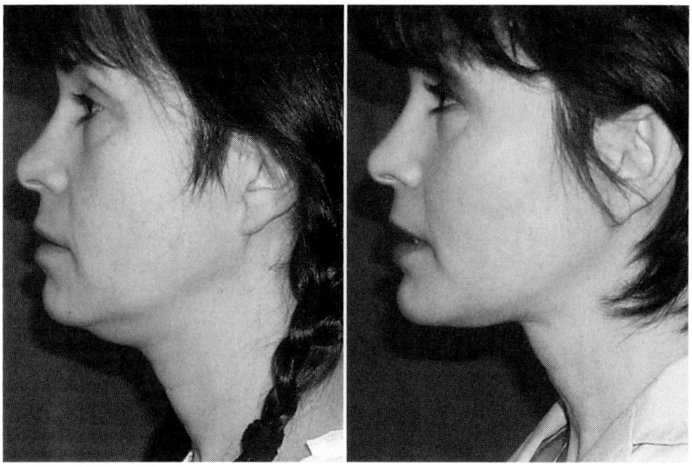

Fig. 5. Before (*left image*) and 4 months after (*right image*) minor superficial liposuction and placement of a small chin implant on a 41-year-old woman.

nerve injury is most commonly transient. If this sequela occurs and persists for over 2 weeks, then consideration may be given to Botox injection to the opposite side to improve symmetry while the nerve recovers. Hyperpigmentation can be managed by hydroquinone 4% twice daily or kojic acid. Skin irregularities are difficult to manage after fibrosis has occurred. Early recognition should prompt the surgeon to have the patient perform vigorous massage daily and return to the office weekly for external ultrasound sessions. Persistent depressed irregularities may be improved with serial fat grafting. If this procedure is unsuccessful, then undermining with face-lift techniques and skin excision may be required in difficult cases.

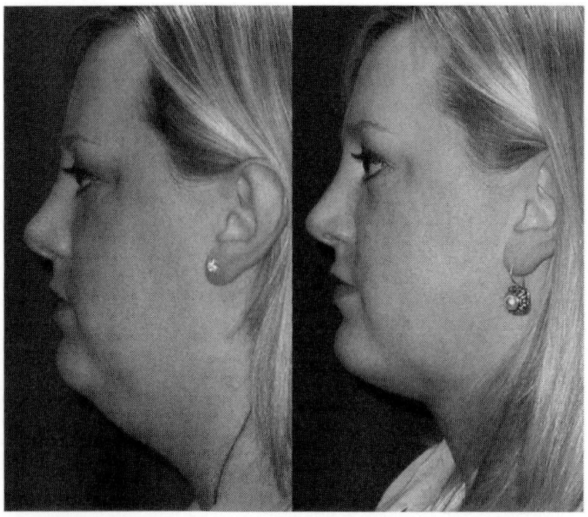

Fig. 6. Before (*left image*) and 1 month after (*right image*) isolated preplatysmal liposuction on a 29-year-old woman.

Submentoplasty

As discussed earlier in the section on patient selection, the patient who has platysmal banding, subplatysmal fat deposits, and submental cutis laxis is likely a candidate for submentoplasty. Many times, submentoplasty is done in conjunction with a rhytidectomy. When there is not significant jowling or when the patient does not desire a more involved procedure, submentoplasty in isolation may be considered.

Anatomy

The important anatomic considerations in the neck include the platysma muscle, the hyoid bone, the anterior jugular veins, the submandibular gland, the facial artery and vein, the marginal mandibular nerve, and the prominence of the thyroid cartilage. The platysma muscle is a quadrangular muscle, with its origin at the fascia of the pectoralis major and its insertion above the inferior border of the mandible, blending with the muscles of facial expression, especially depressor anguli oris. Based on cadaver dissections, the platysma muscle decussates in the midline most of the time. When there is no decussation or poor decussation in the midline, however, the deep fat of the neck can herniate, increasing submental fullness.

In the midline of the neck, the anterior jugular veins are often encountered (Fig. 7). The anterior jugular vein usually begins in the suprahyoid region through a confluence of superficial veins or arises

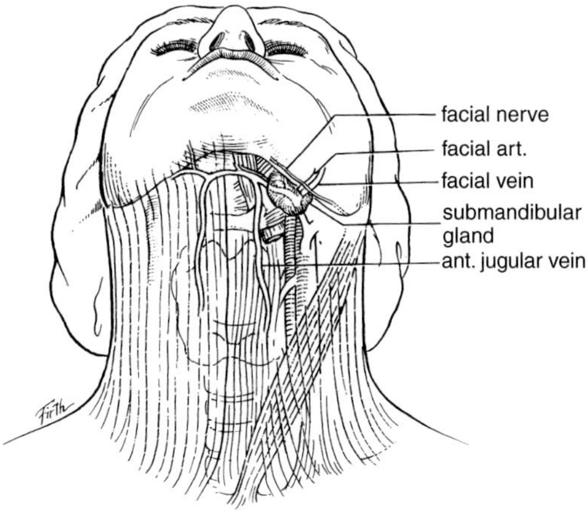

Fig. 7. Commonly encountered anatomic structures during submentoplasty include the anterior jugular veins, submandibular gland, and the facial artery, vein, and nerve. art., artery; ant., anterior.

more laterally from the retromandibular or facial vein [32]. It has variable connections with the facial vein or internal jugular vein. These vessels can create significant bleeding during submentoplasty. The hyoid bone serves as the landmark for backcutting the platysma if planned. The position of the hyoid bone ultimately determines the result that can be achieved with submentoplasty. A low- and anterior-positioned hyoid makes it difficult to get a well-defined cervicomental angle. Often, a chin implant can be used to camouflage this problem by giving the illusion that there is a more acute angle.

Laterally, the facial artery, vein, and nerve and the submandibular gland may be encountered if the surgeon elects to backcut the platysma and perform submuscular undermining. If care is not taken when backcutting the platysma muscle, these structures can be injured (see Fig. 7). In addition, if needed, it is possible to intentionally resect a superficial portion of the submandibular gland through a submental incision to treat submandibular gland ptosis. This resection should be performed with caution because of the increased risk of nerve injury and significant bleeding.

Technique

There have been many techniques described to manage the neck during submentoplasty [14,33–42]. The following techniques describe how the authors typically perform this operation. The technique is varied based on the patient's anatomy.

Situation 1: thin or normal neck, excess fat, submental cutis laxis, with or without platysmal banding or laxity

When a patient has at least fair skin tone and no platysmal banding, he or she may benefit from liposuction alone. If there is any platysmal banding, then platysmaplasty is needed.

First, tumescent anesthesia is used to insufflate approximately 150 mL for an average-sized neck. The mixture that the authors use is 500 mL normal saline, 30 mL lidocaine 2%, plus 1.5 mg epinephrine. A 2- to 3-cm submental incision is made in the natural submental crease. If the patient has a low hyoid position and a chin implant is planned, then the incision is made posterior to the submental crease (Fig. 8). In this way, the incision does not become visible because the chin implant results in the incision appearing more anterior. The dissection is carried down to the level of the platysma with a needle-point cautery.

The authors do not perform liposuction first when doing a platysmaplasty because they believe that it is essential to maintain an even thickness of superficial fat attached to the dermis. Thus, when the skin is redraped, there is less chance of an uneven appearance and skin rippling. Face-lift scissors are used to undermine the skin, leaving an even layer of subdermal fat. The dissection is carried inferiorly as far as the lower border of the thyroid cartilage and laterally to the posterior border of the mandible [43]. Wide skin undermining is necessary to allow proper skin redraping after treatment of the deep tissues has been addressed. Inadequate skin undermining leads to bunching after midline plication of the platysma.

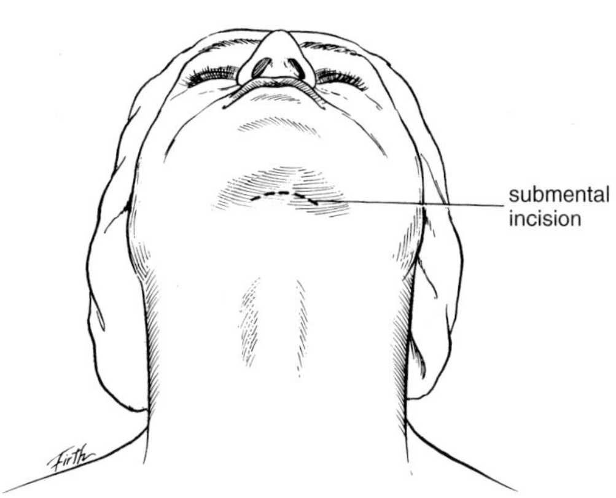

Fig. 8. Incision for submentoplasty is made in the submental crease. If a simulataneous chin implant is planned, then the incision should be made posterior to the submental crease so that it is not visible postoperatively.

A flat spatulated cannula can then be used to perform liposuction on the fat overlying the platysma under direct vision. A lighted Aufricht retractor improves visualization through the small submental incision. Any excess submental fat is then resected. A Kelly clamp or large hemostat is placed in the midline to hold the platysma and fat while a needle-point cautery or scissors are used to resect it (Fig. 9). It is at this point that the anterior jugular veins may be encountered. Proper hemostasis must be achieved; otherwise, it is very difficult to complete the operation properly and there is a greater chance of postoperative hematoma.

After resecting the midline fat, the anterior borders of the platysma and the hyoid bone are identified. The platysma is backcut beginning at the level of the hyoid bone (see Fig. 9). The backcut is carried back an average of 5 to 7 cm, with the cut staying parallel with the inferior border of the mandible and well below the inferior extent of the submandibular gland. When making this incision through platysma, care should be taken to not injure the facial vessels or nerve. The platysma is undermined superior to the area backcut (Fig. 10). When submandibular gland ptosis or gland enlargement is recognized, the authors often manage this by resecting the superficial portion of the gland with the needle-point cautery. This procedure is difficult to do and not recommended for the novice. Bleeding can be encountered that is difficult to control from such a small incision with poor access.

After mobilizing the platysma bilaterally, a corset platysmaplasty is performed. The authors use a running 2-0 Vicryl (Ethicon Inc., Somerville, NJ) suture to do this (Fig. 11). The inferior platysma edges are

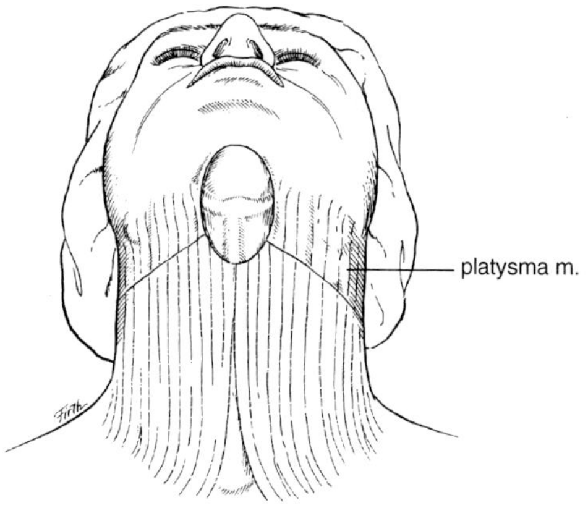

Fig. 10. The platysma muscle is backcut at the level of the hyoid bone, paralleling the inferior border of the mandible. m, muscle.

plicated at the midline to the fascia over the hyoid bone. When a chin implant is to be used to camouflage a poor cervicomental angle related to low hyoid position, it is placed at this time (Figs. 12 and 13). Dissection is carried to the periosteum of the mandible in the midline. A subperiosteal pocket is created at the lower border of the mandible. A solid silicone implant is placed into this pocket. It is secured to the periosteum of the inferior border of the mandible with a single 4-0 Vicryl suture [44]. After ensuring strict hemostasis, the skin is closed with 4-0 monocryl deep and 5-0 plain gut suture on the skin.

A dressing is placed using Reston foam 1563L (3M Medical-Surgical) and a Coban (3M Medical-Surgical) head wrap, worn for 24 hours. When the patient returns the next postoperative day, the wrap is

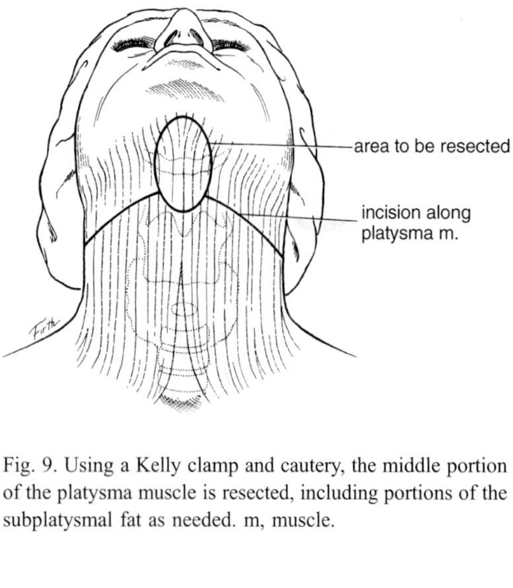

Fig. 9. Using a Kelly clamp and cautery, the middle portion of the platysma muscle is resected, including portions of the subplatysmal fat as needed. m, muscle.

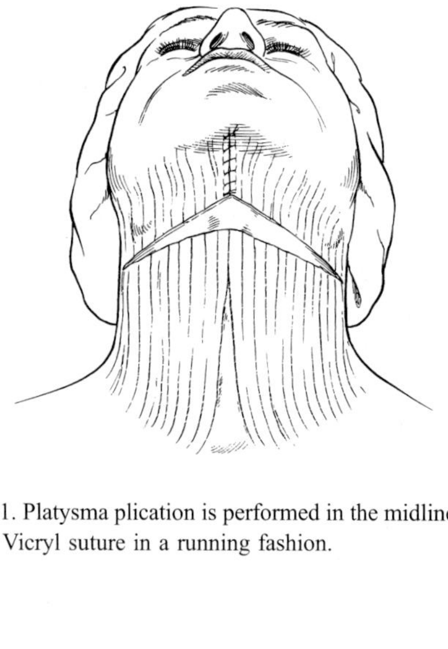

Fig. 11. Platysma plication is performed in the midline using a 2-0 Vicryl suture in a running fashion.

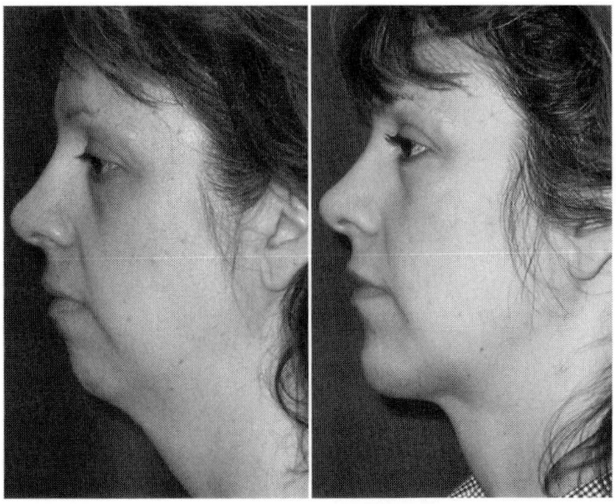

Fig. 12. Before (*left image*) and 4 months after (*right image*) submentoplasty and chin implant placement on a 44-year-old woman who has an anterior preoperative hyoid position.

removed and the patient wears a compression garment such as a face-lift bra. This face-lift bra is to be worn as much as possible, day and night, during the first week. After 1 week, the patient is to wear the garment only at night for 2 more weeks.

Situation 2: thick/obese neck, excess fat, submental cutis laxis, with or without platysmal banding or laxity

The procedure is performed in the same manner as in situation 1, with the following modifications. First, aggressive resection of subplatysmal fat is often performed. Care must be taken to do this resection evenly. The subplatysmal fat can be directly excised with scissors or cautery following elevation of the platysma on either side of midline using a lighted retractor.

Second, although the platysma is backcut in the same manner as in situation 1, a corset suture may not be placed. Instead, a greater portion of the platysma above the hyoid is resected (Figs. 14 and 15). The rationale for vigorous resection of platysma along with pre- and subplatysmal fat in a patient with a very heavy neck is the need to debulk as much as possible to see a significant improvement. These patients are difficult to operate on due to their thick tissue planes and require special treatment. When this resection is not done properly, a cobra neck deformity can result, which is commonly seen after vigorous fat removal from the submentum along with anterior platysmal resection with poor reapproximation of the residual platysmal edges during midline plication.

If anterior plication is to be done in this group of patients, a very clean and thick deep plane flap must be elevated and advanced to the hyoid under very little tension (Figs. 16 and 17). Although the plication is necessary to avoid a skeletonized appearance in the patient with an average or thin neck, it is often not necessary in a patient with an obese neck and can even compromise the end result [45]. An anterior plication, if performed at all in these patients, must be very secure to prevent breakdown that may render postoperative paramedian bands from the cut platysmal edges. With special care to create a uniform layer of deep fat and neck musculature in the very obese neck, however, resection of the platysma and subplatysmal fat often leads to a longer lasting and maximized result in this more difficult patient population. When performing major tissue debulking (of fat and muscle), it is critical to leave a smooth and relatively thick layer of fat on the underside of the skin flap along with a uniform contour of the residual deep tissues in the neck. Strict hemostasis is also a must. Although this technique is challenging because of the small incision, it can give wonderful results when diligently performed in this difficult subset of patients.

Situation 3: submentoplasty with face-lift

A face-lift is necessary when the patient wants significant elevation of sagging jowls or other tissues above the mandibular border along with neck improvement. When a face-lift is to be performed, the authors may perform liposuction before elevating the skin flap. Doing so facilitates the dissection. If an aggressive submentoplasty is to be performed, then no liposuction is performed in the submental region before the dissection. The reason for this is so that a very clean surgical field can be obtained to perform

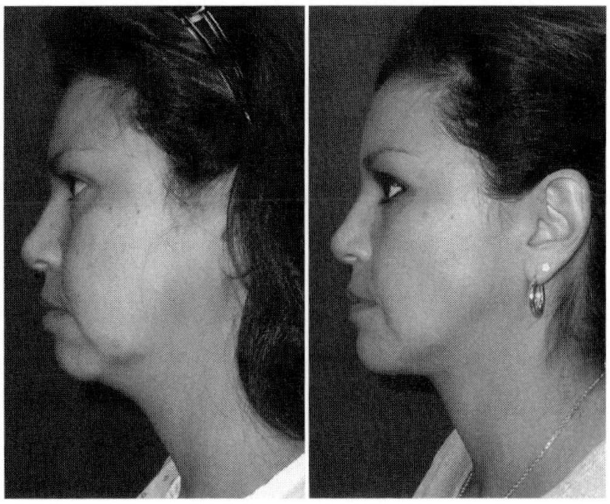

Fig. 13. Before (*left image*) and 6 months after (*right image*) submentoplasty and chin implant placement on a 45-year-old woman who has a normal preoperative hyoid position.

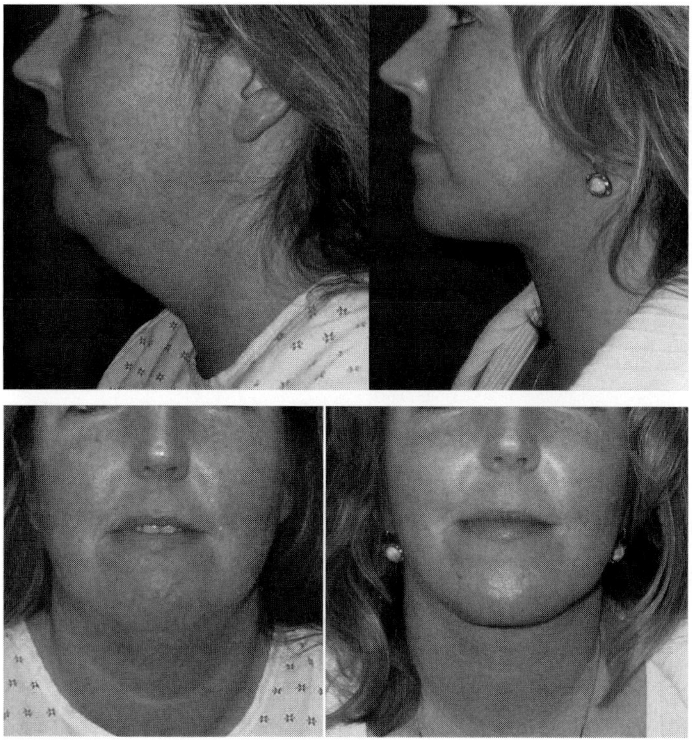

Fig. 14. Before (*upper- and lower-left images*) and 2 months after (*upper- and lower-right images*) aggressive submentoplasty with direct subplatysmal fat excision an platysmal muscle resection on a 37-year-old woman.

the submentoplasty. After the submentoplasty is performed, a large, flat liposuction cannula is used under direct vision to clean off any excess fat from the platysma. A large, flat liposuction cannula may also used to clean off excess fat from the SMAS after the rhytidectomy flap is elevated. This open liposuction technique allows the operator to directly visualize areas that require further liposuction to obtain smooth skin contours after the flap is redraped and sutured.

Although the authors believe that a submentoplasty is almost always a necessity when simultaneously performing a face-lift, it is not necessarily performed by many face-lift surgeons [46]. There are two prevalent reasons for not performing a simultaneous submentoplasty with a face-lift. First, some surgeons believe that it is not worth the time because the posterior SMAS pull alone improves the anterior neck tissues. Of course, performing posterior imbrication alone may do well for some necks initially, but may ultimately lead to relapse of tissue laxity in the anterior neck 4 to 6 months following the face-lift. Second, midline platysmal plication may compromise some of the elevation that could otherwise be obtained in the jowl region because the anterior pull is partially competing with the SMAS elevation from the face-lift. Attaining less jowl elevation may occur when doing submentoplasty with a short-flap technique, but it does not seem to be a problem when combining a submentoplasty with a long-flap face-lift technique. The goal in any cosmetic rejuve-

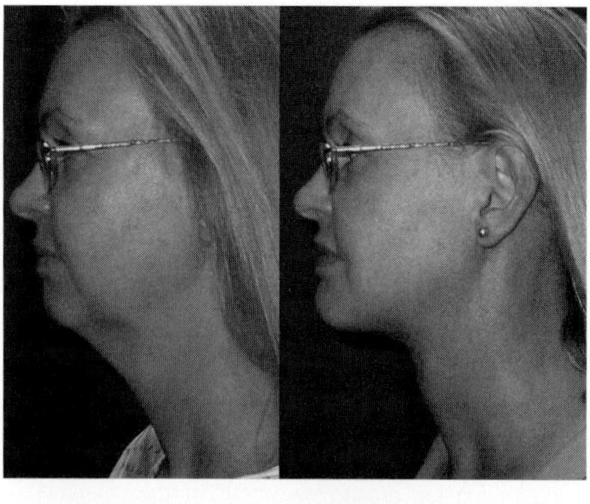

Fig. 15. Before (*left image*) and 5 weeks after (*right image*) submentoplasty with platysmal backcutting and partial resection along with chin implant on a 43-year-old woman.

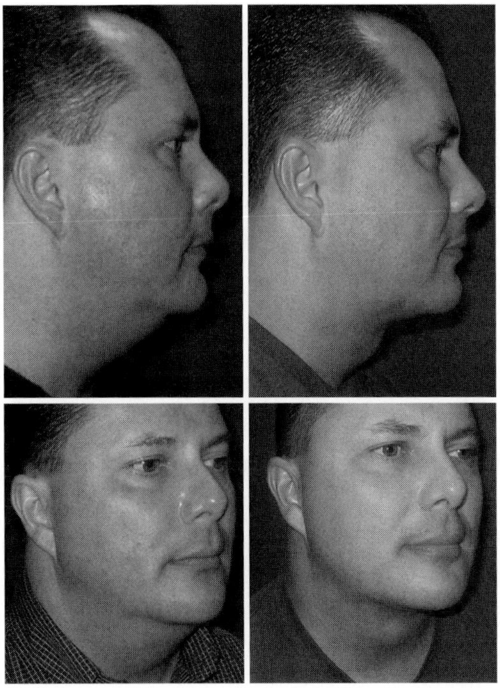

Fig. 16. Before (*upper- and lower-left images*) and 7 months after (*upper- and lower-right images*) an aggressive submentoplasty (subplatysmal fat excision and horizontal platysmal backcutting with anterior plication) on a 43-year-old man.

nation procedure is a more youthful appearance that is natural and long lasting. Combining an anterior platysmalplasty with a face-lift is usually necessary to achieve the latter.

Partial submandibular gland resection

This technique is used principally for patients who have had previous neck liposuction or face-lifting and now notice their submandibular glands bulging for the first time [47,48]. Patients typically are worried because they are unsure of the etiology of their recently noticed lateral neck bulge. An astute surgeon may occasionally diagnosis enlarged or ptotic submandibular glands before an initial neck surgery. It is unfortunate that this condition is usually seen as a side effect subsequent to a cosmetic procedure. Over-resection of fat may contribute to the problem. Regardless, the options are limited. Simply reassuring the patient after a procedure may be adequate, especially if this condition was discussed as a risk during the preoperative visit. Surgical treatments are available but have a mixed history of success combined with a higher than average complication rate, even with experienced surgeons.

The authors' particular technique has been used for just over 3 years and in 48 patients who have primary or secondary submandibular gland enlargement or ptosis. The procedure is performed solely through a submental crease incision with a long skin flap, followed by subplatysmal muscle elevation beginning on either side of the midline. Backcutting the platysma horizontally at the level of the hyoid is also required. Excellent visualization is critical, along with an expert knowledge of the local anatomy and judicious use of electrocautery. The authors' technique is simply a modification of the submentoplasty technique previously discussed in the "Submentoplasty/Technique" section for thin- or normal-framed patients with average neck problems. The only difference is that following elevation of the platysmal flap, a small perforation is created with needle-tip cautery through the cervical fascia that covers the lowest and most anterior portion of the submandibular gland, which is easily seen as a large bulge beneath the elevated submuscular flap (Fig. 18).

After it is exposed, the submandibular gland is grasped with a long forceps to elevate the excessive gland from its pocket, whereby it can be amputated slowly with electrocautery. Caution must be taken to avoid deep transection of the gland while working through a distant and small anterior incision because bleeding from even a small branch of the facial artery can be difficult to deal with from this limited access. Closure of the cervical fascia perforation over the residual gland with 2-0 Vicryl can be performed with a single interrupted suture. The closure of fascia over

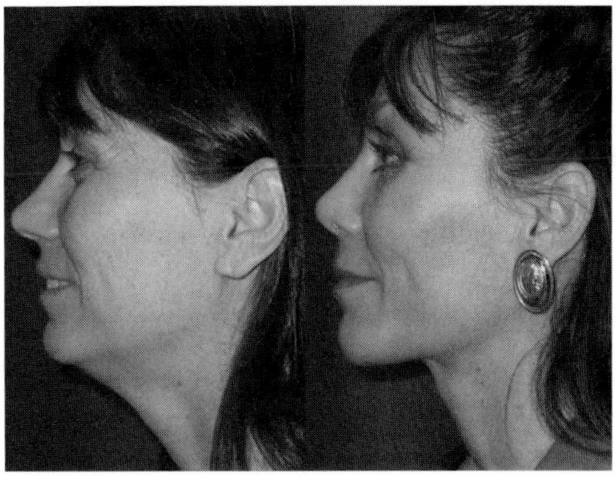

Fig. 17. Before (*left image*) and 2 months after (*right image*) isolated submentoplasty using a horizontal backcut and anterior plication of the platysma on a 49-year-old woman.

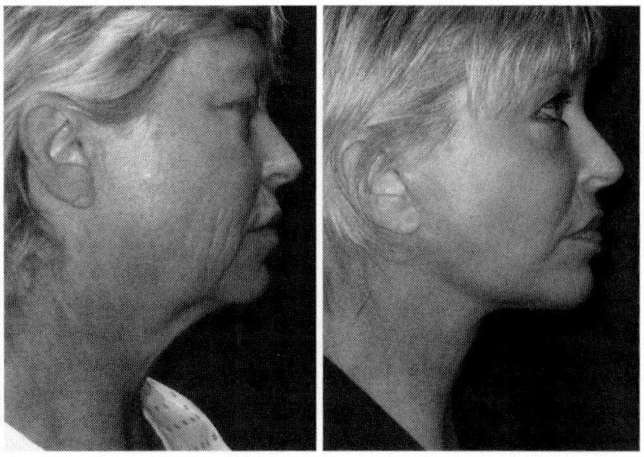

Fig. 18. Before (*left image*) and 3 months after (*right image*) lower face-lift combined with submentoplasty and simultaneous partial submandibular gland resection on a 57-year-old woman.

the gland is not absolutely necessary but may decrease the chance of postoperative hematoma, sialoceles, or recurrent gland ptosis. This procedure is for experienced surgeons and has a definite learning curve that may require aborted treatment the first few times the technique is attempted. It has been the authors' experience, however, that partial resection is a viable option for the appropriate patient and the results far exceed any previous sling techniques.

Complications

In general, the complications following submentoplasty closely resemble those following neck liposuction alone. For the most part, these complications (dermal injury with postoperative indurations, skin irregularities, prolonged swelling, seromas, hematomas, sialoceles, transient and permanent injury of the marginal mandibular nerve, and post-inflammatory hyperpigmentation) are treated as previously discussed under the "Liposuction" section in this article.

Due to the fact that a large subcutaneous skin flap must be elevated for most submentoplasty techniques, the large dead space increases the chance for postoperative fluid accumulation (eg, hematoma, seroma, or sialocele). Because the incidence of postoperative hematoma is much higher with submentoplasty than with liposuction alone and often much larger in volume, treatment may require more aggressive therapy than simple aspiration. The authors' hematoma rate for isolated submentoplasty equals their rate for hematoma following face-lift surgery, which is 3% for small hematomas requiring aspiration only and 1% for large hematomas requiring surgical drainage. Open surgical drainage and wound exploration must be considered for any large hematomas (greater than 60 mL) or for any with obvious signs of continued hemorrhage. Even when serial aspiration can be used alone, the fluid often needs to be drained multiple times every other day as long as the total aspirate continues to decrease in volume at each visit. Pressure wraps are continued until the reaccumulation stops.

Hematomas usually occur within the first 24 hours. Often, they occur a few hours after the anesthetic wears off and the patient experiences pain and an increase in their blood pressure along with local rebound vasodilation at the surgical site. Early treatment is critical. Without adequate and early treatment, hematomas can result in hyperpigmentation and rippling of the skin secondary to subdermal scarring. Induration will also be much worse. Skin slough is generally not a problem in patients undergoing an isolated submentoplasty but could be a potential dreadful sequela following an untreated expanding hematoma. Aggressive and early management is needed along with frequent and close follow-up appointments. Early external ultrasound therapy along with local massage by the patient can significantly decrease postoperative induration.

Sialoceles, although relatively uncommon (less than 0.5%), are certainly more frequent after aggressive submentoplasty or deep-plane face-lift techniques than after neck liposuction alone. As discussed previously in this article, treatment for sialoceles after submentoplasty is the same as after liposuction, but it must be realized that a sialocele from the parotid has much higher fluid collections, requires more frequent aspirations, and may take up to 1 month to fully resolve. Sialoceles rarely require surgical management unless the volume does not continue to decrease with each aspiration or the overlying skin integrity is compromised.

Finally, an unfortunate complication is adhesion of the platysma or digastric muscles to the overlying skin when excess fat has been removed through liposuction or surgical technique. This adhesion can result in a rippled or uneven appearance to the skin. Over-resection of deep tissues may also produce an unsightly, skeletonized appearance that is difficult to treat and should be avoided if at all possible. The authors believe that a skeletonized appearance can be prevented by raising the skin flap first to maintain an even thickness of fat. When liposuction is done first, this problem is more likely to be encountered. If this problem occurs, then treatment may require serial fat grafting or occasional skin elevation and redraping.

Summary

Poor neck contour is a frequent complaint of patients. Often, the most appropriate procedure is a cervicofacial rhytidectomy; however, there are instances in which a less aggressive and perhaps minimally invasive procedure can provide good esthetic results. The patient with isolated submental fat deposits with good skin tone and minimal platysmal laxity may benefit from liposuction alone. Even patients who refuse a face-lift and have significant platysmal banding and laxity can have dramatic improvement with submentoplasty alone. Of course, patients must be informed that they may require additional procedures if these isolated techniques are not completely effective in treating their problem. Limitations aside, isolated neck liposuction with or without associated submentoplasty can be a superb minimally invasive cosmetic procedure. The appropriate patient will appreciate the improved neck appearance coupled with a decreased downtime compared with traditional neck or face-lift techniques.

References

[1] Dayan SH, Bagal A, Tardy Jr ME. Targeted solutions in submentoplasty. Facial Plast Surg 2001;17:141.

[2] Guyuron B. Problem neck, hyoid bone, and submental myotomy. Plast Reconstr Surg 1992;90:830.

[3] Ramirez OM, Robertson KM. Comprehensive approach to rejuvenation of the neck. Facial Plast Surg 2001;17:129.

[4] Hetter GP. Improved results with closed facial suction. Clin Plast Surg 1989;16:319.

[5] Hoefflin SM. Anatomy of the platysma and lip depressor muscles. A simplified mnemonic approach. Dermatol Surg 1998;24:1225.

[6] Adamson PA, Cormier R, Tropper GJ, et al. Cervicofacial liposuction: results and controversies. J Otolaryngol 1990;19:267.

[7] Bach DE, Newhouse RF, Boice GW. Simultaneous orthognathic surgery and cervicomental liposuction. Clinical and survey results. Oral Surg Oral Med Oral Pathol 1991;71:262.

[8] Bank DE, Perez MI. Skin retraction after liposuction in patients over the age of 40. Dermatol Surg 1999; 25:673.

[9] Chrisman BB. Liposuction with facelift surgery. Dermatol Clin 1990;8:501.

[10] Daher JC, Cosac OM, Domingues S. Face-lift: the importance of redefining facial contours through facial liposuction. Ann Plast Surg 1988;21:1.

[11] Dedo DD. Liposuction of the head and neck. Otolaryngol Head Neck Surg 1987;97:591.

[12] Goodstein WA. Superficial liposculpture of the face and neck. Plast Reconstr Surg 1996;98:988.

[13] Grotting JC, Beckenstein MS. Cervicofacial rejuvenation using ultrasound-assisted lipectomy. Plast Reconstr Surg 2001;107:847.

[14] Jacob CI, Berkes BJ, Kaminer MS. Liposuction and surgical recontouring of the neck: a retrospective analysis. Dermatol Surg 2000;26:625.

[15] O'Ryan F, Schendel S, Poor D. Submental-submandibular suction lipectomy: indications and surgical technique. Oral Surg Oral Med Oral Pathol 1989;67:117.

[16] Gryskiewicz JM. Submental suction-assisted lipectomy without platysmaplasty: pushing the (skin) envelope to avoid a face lift for unsuitable candidates. Plast Reconstr Surg 2003;112:1393.

[17] Hanke CW, Bullock S, Bernstein G. Current status of tumescent liposuction in the United States. National survey results. Dermatol Surg 1996;22:595.

[18] Hanke CW, Coleman III WP. Morbidity and mortality related to liposuction. Questions and answers. Dermatol Clin 1999;17:899.

[19] Housman TS, Lawrence N, Mellen BG, et al. The safety of liposuction: results of a national survey. Dermatol Surg 2002;28:971.

[20] Jones BM, Grover R. Reducing complications in cervicofacial rhytidectomy by tumescent infiltration: a comparative trial evaluating 678 consecutive face lifts. Plast Reconstr Surg 2004;113:398.

[21] Klein JA. History of tumescent liposuction. In: Klein J, editor. Tumescent technique: Tumescent anesthesia & microcannular liposuction, vol. 1. St. Louis (MO): Mosby; 2000. p. 4.

[22] Klein JA. The tumescent technique. Anesthesia and modified liposuction technique. Dermatol Clin 1990; 8:425.

[23] Ostad A, Kageyama N, Moy RL. Tumescent anesthesia with a lidocaine dose of 55 mg/kg is safe for liposuction. Dermatol Surg 1996;22:921.

[24] Rao RB, Ely SF, Hoffman RS. Deaths related to liposuction. N Engl J Med 1999;340:1471.

[25] Klein JA. Tumescent technique for regional anesthesia permits lidocaine doses of 35 mg/kg for liposuction. J Dermatol Surg Oncol 1990;16:248.

[26] LaTrenta GS, Talmore M. Tumescent cervicofacial rhytidectomy. Perspect Plast Surg 2001;15:47.

[27] Rubin JP, Bierman C, Rosow CE, et al. The tumescent technique: the effect of high tissue pressure and dilute epinephrine on absorption of lidocaine. Plast Reconstr Surg 1999;103:990.

[28] Coldiron B. Office surgical incidents: 19 months of Florida data. Dermatol Surg 2002;28:710.

[29] Burk III RW, Guzman-Stein G, Vasconez LO. Lidocaine and epinephrine levels in tumescent technique liposuction. Plast Reconstr Surg 1996;97:1379.

[30] Klein JA. Anesthetic formulation of tumescent solutions. Dermatol Clin 1999;17:751.

[31] Dillerud E. Suction lipoplasty: a report on complications, undesired results, and patient satisfaction based on 3511 procedures. Plast Reconstr Surg 1991;88:239.

[32] Hollinshead HW. The neck. In: Anatomy for surgeons: the head and neck. vol. 1. Philadelphia: Lippincott-Raven; 1982. p. 467–70.
[33] Feldman JJ. Corset platysmaplasty. Clin Plast Surg 1992;19:369.
[34] Feldman JJ. Corset platysmaplasty. Plast Reconstr Surg 1990;85:333.
[35] Fuente del Campo A. Midline platysma muscular overlap for neck restoration. Plast Reconstr Surg 1998; 102:1710.
[36] Giampapa VC, Di Bernardo BE. Neck recontouring with suture suspension and liposuction: an alternative for the early rhytidectomy candidate. Aesthetic Plast Surg 1995;19:217.
[37] Jasin ME. Submentoplasty as an isolated rejuvenative procedure for the neck. Arch Facial Plast Surg 2003; 5:180.
[38] Kamer FM. Isolated platysmaplasty: a useful procedure but with important limitations. Arch Facial Plast Surg 2003;5:184.
[39] Kamer FM, Frankel AS. Isolated submentoplasty. A limited approach to the aging neck. Arch Otolaryngol Head Neck Surg 1997;123:66.
[40] Kamer FM, Lefkoff LA. Submental surgery. A graduated approach to the aging neck. Arch Otolaryngol Head Neck Surg 1991;117:40.
[41] Knize DM. Limited incision submental lipectomy and platysmaplasty. Plast Reconstr Surg 1998; 101:473.
[42] Knize DM. Limited incision submental lipectomy and platysmaplasty. Plast Reconstr Surg 2004; 113:1275.
[43] Ramirez OM. Cervicoplasty: nonexcisional anterior approach. Plast Reconstr Surg 1997;99:1576.
[44] Louis PJ, Cuzalina LA. Alloplastic augmentation of the face. Atlas Oral Maxillofac Surg Clin N Am 2000;8:127.
[45] Knipper P, Mitz V, Maladry D, et al. Is it necessary to suture the platysma muscles on the midline to improve the cervical profile? An anatomic study using 20 cadavers. Ann Plast Surg 1997;39:566.
[46] Perkins SW, Gibson FB. Use of submentoplasty to enhance cervical recontouring in face-lift surgery. Arch Otolaryngol Head Neck Surg 1993;119:179.
[47] de Pina DP, Quinta WC. Aesthetic resection of the submandibular salivary gland. Plast Reconstr Surg 1991;88:779.
[48] Singer DP, Sullivan PK. Submandibular gland I: an anatomic evaluation and surgical approach to submandibular gland resection for facial rejuvenation. Plast Reconstr Surg 2003;112:1150.

ELSEVIER
SAUNDERS

Oral Maxillofacial Surg Clin N Am 17 (2005) 99 – 109

ORAL AND
MAXILLOFACIAL
SURGERY CLINICS
of North America

Autologous Fat Augmentation for Addressing Facial Volume Loss

Suzan Obagi, MD

Cosmetic Surgery and Skin Health Center, University of Pittsburgh Medical Center, 1603 Carmody Court, Suite 103, Pittsburgh, PA, 15143, USA

Fat transplantation has been the subject of much interest and great debate over the years. As we begin to analyze the long-term results of traditional "lifting" procedures such as face-lifts, eye-lifts, and brow-lifts, we realize that we have achieved a "tighter" and "lifted" appearance for our patients without truly achieving a rejuvenated look. Dr. Sam Hamra [1] elegantly shows this concept of lifting without achieving rejuvenation in a study in which he critically evaluated the long-term results of his deep-plane rhytidectomy. He found that he was able to achieve short-term improvement of the nasolabial fold but that after a few years, this result diminished considerably. At the same time, the deep-plane face-lift failed to achieve rejuvenation of the midface/periorbital region as would have been evidenced by a shortened vertical height of the periorbital region. Although these findings may not become evident until years after a procedure, if a surgeon fails to critically analyze his/her results, then these findings may not make it into the scientific literature.

By analytically evaluating surgical results and by better understanding the mechanisms by which the face ages, a renewed focus has been seen in volume restoration during facial rejuvenation. This renewed interest, however, has also revived some of the controversies that plague fat augmentation.

There is no argument that if one was to search for a substance that fulfills the criteria of an ideal filler, fat would win. Autologous fat is nonimmunogenic, available in relative abundance, is a living tissue, and easily conforms to the properties of the area into which it is injected.

Considering these advantages, one wonders why fat transplantation remains such a hotly debated subject. Academic meetings and peer-reviewed articles are replete with examples of the debate that ensues when the discussion focuses on the long-term survival of fat grafts. Because there are numerous techniques being used to harvest, prepare, and inject fat grafts, it is not surprising that the results achieved vary from surgeon to surgeon. As surgeons begin to review their long-term results, however, it seems that there are similarities between the techniques that seem to yield the best longevity of the grafts. These similarities are the focus of this article. The author presents the technique used in over 200 patients over the past 4 years.

Facial volume loss

The aging face shows characteristic changes, many of which are solely attributed to the effects of gravity on skin, muscle, and fat. Indeed, a number of previous studies have focused on the concept of ptosis secondary to gravity as the predominant factor in midfacial aging, and techniques have been developed based on this concept to excise skin, fat, and fascia while resuspending muscles. A close analysis of the results achieved by these surgeries shows that although the patient indeed looks tighter and lifted, the patient does not necessarily look rejuvenated. This result indicates that ptosis remains only one of a multitude of changes that contribute to the stigmata of the aging face.

E-mail address: obagi@imap.pitt.edu

1042-3699/05/$ – see front matter
doi:10.1016/j.coms.2004.11.001

Although the scientific literature has covered the bony changes that take place over time, this research is largely ignored when planning aesthetic procedures. Yet, to restore the youthful look of a patient, the importance of the bony changes in the midface must be recognized.

A well-designed CT study showed that the lower midfacial skeleton becomes retrusive with age relative to the upper face [2]. In addition, this retrusion occurs at a point below the nasolabial fold, suggesting that relative maxillary retrusion is a factor in the development of the nasolabial fold. These investigators further speculated that the skeletal remodeling of the anterior maxillary wall allows the soft tissues to be repositioned downward, thereby accentuating the nasojugal fold and malar mound.

Furthermore, an excellent study by Gosain et al [3] on the pathogenesis of the nasolabial fold showed a combined effect of ptosis and fat/skin hypertrophy. The investigators used MRI technology to evaluate the midcheek/nasolabial fold in young women (16–30 years old) versus older women (>60 years old) (Fig. 1). Results showed that older women had a relatively increased thickness of the midportion of the malar fat pad and overlying skin. They found no significant change in length or projection of the levator labii superioris muscle between young and old subjects. Their observation that thickness of the upper portion of the fat pad did not decrease while thickness of the midportion of the fat pad increased indicates that a redistribution of the cheek fat (ptosis) and increased volume of the fat (hypertrophy) may have contributed to deepening of the nasolabial fold in old subjects.

Even with the bony and soft-tissue changes mentioned previously, one cannot fully account for all the changes in the aging face. Therefore, one must look at the soft-tissue volume distribution changes that take place from youth to old age. Surgeons who perform a great deal of volume restoration surgeries have shed insight into the morphologic changes that take place over the years [4,5].

Donofrio [4] described the three-dimensional young face as being defined by three primary arcs: (1) lateral cheek projection from the tarsus down to the lower face, (2) along the jawline on each side from the lateral mandible to the mentum, and (3) on the forehead and continuing into the convexity of the brow. There also are a number of secondary arcs. In contrast, the aging face shows dramatic demarcation of the various cosmetic subunits. The primary arcs now become disrupted and replaced with "broken, wavy, or concave" shapes. The loss of volume in these regions creates a relative excess of skin. In addition, Donofrio [4] mentioned a distinct subset of older patients that develops hypertrophy of the fat in certain regions of the face: submental, jowl, lateral nasolabial fold, lateral labiomental crease, and the lateral malar areas. In these patients, she advocates liposuction while lipofilling the atrophied areas.

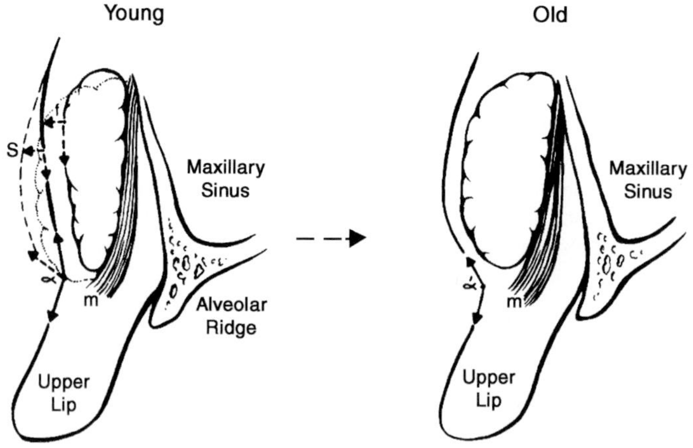

Fig. 1. Summary of directional changes from young to old subjects of the soft tissues within the medial portion of the check mass in repose. In old subjects, thickness of the cheek fat pad (f) and skin (S) is significantly increased at midaxis, resulting in increased depth of the nasolabial fold and a more acute angle of the nasolabial fold ([α] = angle of nasolabial fold in young subjects; [α'] = angle of nasolabial fold in old subjects). (*From* Gosain AK, Amarante MTJ, Hyde JS, et al. A dynamic analysis of changes in the nasolabial fold using magnetic resonance imaging: implications for facial rejuvenation and facial animation surgery. Plast Reconstr Surg 1996;98(4):631; with permission.)

Coleman [5] suggested that the aging face begins to show more of the fat in the jowls, above the nasolabial folds, and in the eyelids as the surrounding fullness disappears. In addition, the bony skull becomes more noticeable in certain areas as volume is lost.

By combining the information from the studies and the surgeons discussed previously, a model emerges that integrates the hard- and soft-tissue components of midfacial aging. It is only by addressing these changes using volume restoration rather than simply using lifting procedures that surgeons can offer their patients the youthful appearance they desire.

Harvesting techniques

Many factors can affect the harvesting of viable adipocytes, from local anesthetics, harvesting techniques (tissue trauma), and desiccation (prolonged exposure to air), to the preparation of the adipocytes. What is unknown, however, is the exact extent to which adipocytes are harmed by the handling methods. The scientific literature is replete with examples of conflicting studies on these issues.

There is debate over which sites yield the most viable adipocytes, with some surgeons advocating any site for harvesting and other surgeons using only diet-resistant areas. A recent well-designed study in which fat was harvested from four areas per patient (abdomen, flank, medial knee, and thigh) showed no difference in adipocyte viability [6]. Therefore, the most accessible donor site is used. Care is taken to remove fat without causing iatrogenic defects. Accordingly, it is occasionally necessary to select several donor sites, especially in thinner individuals.

Local anesthesia of the donor site can be achieved using a modified Klein's solution of 0.1% to 0.2% lidocaine with epinephrine 1:500,000 to 1:1,000,000 (Table 1). Although lidocaine can affect the metabolic activity of adipocytes (glucose transport, lipolysis, and growth) in-vitro, it seems that this effect is only transitory and that normal metabolic function resumes after the lidocaine is no longer present [7].

Rather than tumescent anesthesia of an area, a wet technique is used. Approximately 120 mL to 200 mL is infiltrated into the tissue using 20-gauge spinal needles. Usually, 1 to 3 mL of anesthetic is used for each milliliter of fat to be aspirated. The solution is allowed to take effect for 5 to 10 minutes to ensure proper analgesia and vasoconstriction.

Harvesting adipocytes in the least traumatic way possible helps increase the number of viable cells available for transplantation. For this reason, the use of a liposuction aspiration machine is discouraged. Manual suction is best achieved by using a 10-mL syringe in which the plunger is withdrawn 1 to 2 mL during the aspiration of the fat. A Coleman 3-mm harvesting cannula (Byron Medical, Tucson, Arizona) is used (Fig. 2). The design of the cannula is such that fat parcels that pass through it can then be easily passed through the 17-gauge infiltrating cannulas and into the recipient site.

An important consideration in fat harvesting is to normalize oncotic pressure by adding 1 to 2 mL of human albumin to the 10-mL syringe before harvesting the fat. Because the use of the modified Klein's solution is hypo-oncotic, the harvested fat will have 1.1 to 1.2 g% protein (normal is 2–4 g%) [8]. Albumin not only normalizes oncotic pressure but also acts to further condense the harvested adipocytes by allowing for greater fluid removal from the cells [9].

If the aspirated fat becomes blood-tinged, then it is important to move away from that area so that the bulk of the aspirated fat is bloodless. When there is too much fluid in the harvested fat, one can wait a few minutes or massage the donor area to allow for resorption of some of the anesthetic fluid before further harvesting.

Table 1
Modified Klein's solutions used to achive local anesthesia

0.2 % Lidocaine, epinephrine 1:500,000	0.1 % Lidocaine, epinephrine 1:500,000
500 cc normal saline 0.9%, sterile	500 cc normal saline 0.9%, sterile
50 cc 2% lidocaine	25 cc 2% lidocaine
1 mL epinephrine 1:1,000	1 mL epinephrine 1:1,000
10 cc sodium bicarbonate	10 cc sodium bicarbonate

Fat processing

The 10-mL syringes of fat are capped and centrifuged in a sterile fashion at 3100 rpm for 2 minutes (Fig. 3). Although there exists controversy over the use of centrifugation [6,10], most surgeons use it to further condense the fat while yielding reproducible results in their patients.

Centrifugation results in three layers in the 10-mL syringe: infranatant (fluid, blood), middle layer (fat), and supranatant (triglycerides, oil) (Fig. 4). The infranatant and supranatant are decanted, and the

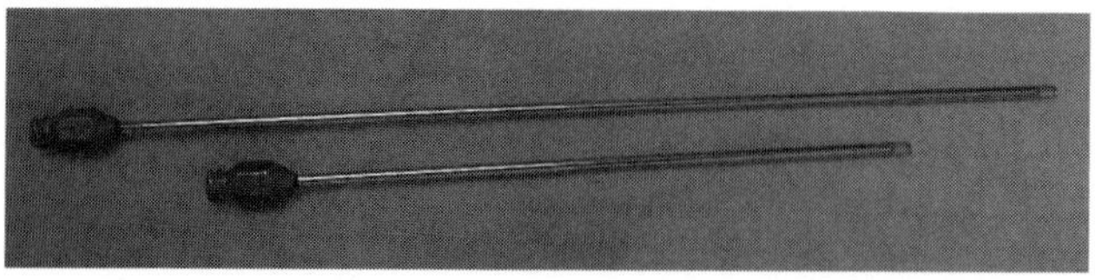

Fig. 2. Coleman Harvesting Cannula (3 mm; Byron Medical).

remaining fat is transferred to 1-mL syringes without the use of any adapters (Fig. 5).

Choosing the best site for graft placement

There is much debate as to where to place the fat grafts for optimal survival [11,12]. Although fat grafts contain viable adipocytes, failure to re-establish a vascular supply at the recipient site causes necrosis and ultimate loss of the grafts. There are several factors to consider when placing the grafts.

The subcutaneous fat at the recipient site is relatively avascular, whereas the muscle and fascia layers contain a richer vascular supply around which fat grafts may survive better. Guerrerosantos et al [12] showed in a rat model that grafted fat (as lipoinjection of thin rolls or as strips) survived best when injected into or around muscle. In the study groups in which the fat was injected subcutaneously, there was no long-term retention of the grafts. In addition, injection of larger volumes of fat resulted in cyst formation with central necrosis.

Although some investigators advocate layering the fat into two to three layers (subcutaneous, muscle, supraperiosteal) [4,5], some advocate only intramuscular placement [13,14]. The author favors a layering technique in which two to three layers of tissue are infiltrated. This technique is based on the fact that there is growing evidence that preadipocytes (stem cells) are present in the harvested fat [15] and may take on the characteristics of the tissue into which they are injected (muscle, fat, cartilage). Therefore, it seems that placement into several tissue layers will only enhance the potential transformation of the preadipocytes into a variety of tissue.

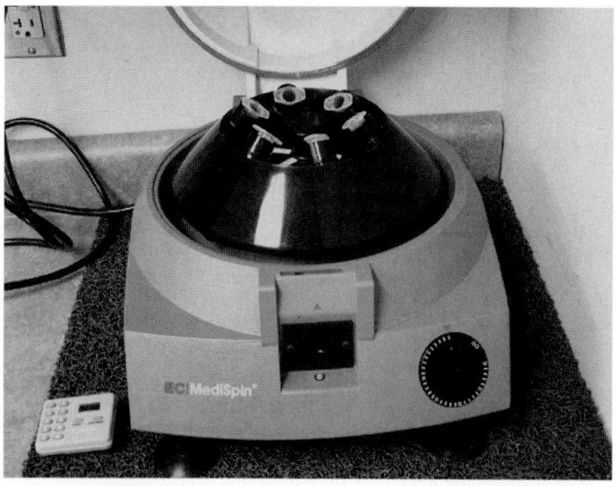

Fig. 3. Syringe caps and centrifuge.

Fat infiltration techniques

Although many surgeons advocate the use of blunt cannulas for infiltrating the fat, some surgeons solely use sharp needles to place the fat in subdermal tunnels [16]. Caution must be taken while using sharp instruments, however, to avoid nerve and vessel injury (see "Complications").

The patient is photographed, consented, and then marked while in an upright position. After the fat is harvested, the face is prepped and draped in a sterile fashion while the assistant prepares the fat. Appropriate nerve blocks are performed by using 1% lidocaine with epinephrine and a 30-gauge 1 inch needle. This step is followed by fanning some of the modified Klein's solution into areas not reached by the

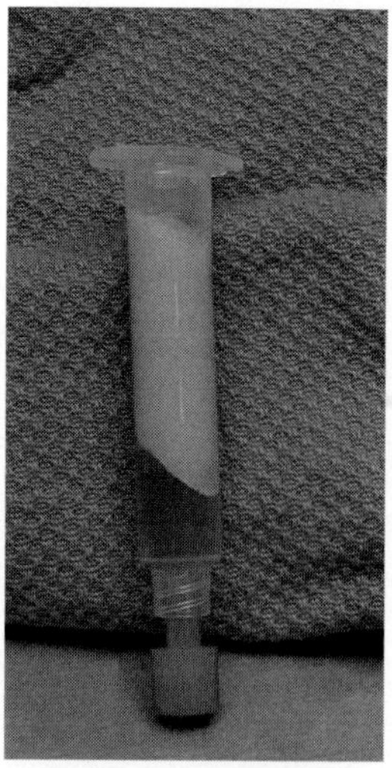

Fig. 4. Centrifuged fat showing three layers: supranatant layer of triglycerides/oil, middle layer of fat, and infranatant (blood, fluid).

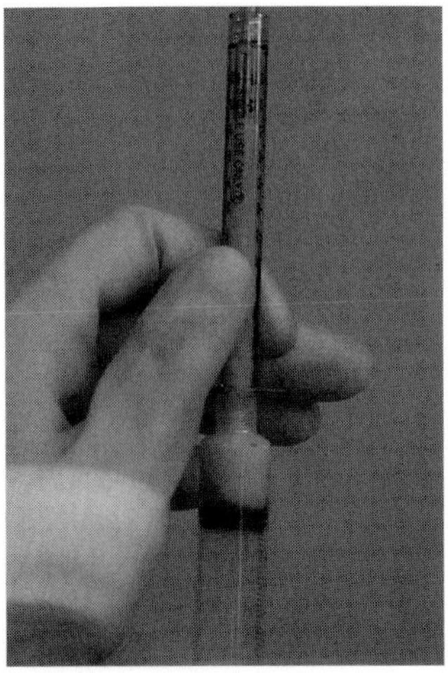

Fig. 5. Transfer of fat from the 10-mL syringe into 1-mL syringes without a luer-to-luer adapter.

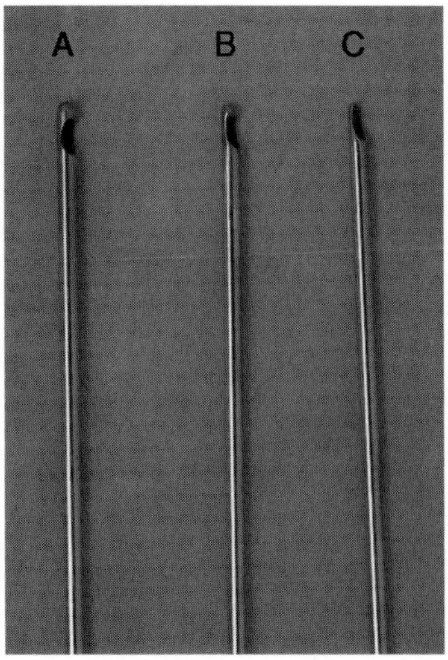

Fig. 7. Coleman cannulas: (*A*) No. 1, most blunt tip; (*B*) No. 2, intermediate tip; (*C*) No. 3, least blunt tip.

nerve blocks using a 25-gauge spinal needle. The assistant holds pressure after each injection to minimize bruising. For both cheeks, for example, 4 to 6 mL of 1% lidocaine with epinephrine is used for the infraorbital, mental, and zygomaticofacial nerve blocks, followed by approximately another 20 mL of 0.2% lidocaine with epinephrine 1:500,000 to anesthetize the lateral cheeks and further anesthetize the chin.

Incision sites are kept at a minimum, with most of the midface and temples reached from one incision at the zygomatic arch, near the lateral orbital rim (Fig. 6). The incision is made with a 16-gauge No-Kor needle (Becton Dickinson, Franklin Lakes, New Jersey). At the conclusion of the procedure, all incisions are closed with a single suture using 6.0 fast-absorbing gut suture.

The 1-mL syringes of fat are infiltrated into different levels by using most commonly a Coleman No. 2 cannula (Fig. 7). Care is taken to infiltrate only 0.05 to 0.1 mL of fat per parcel. This method keeps as much of the surface area of the adipocytes as possible in contact with the surrounding tissue from which they must draw nutrition until they re-establish their vascular supply.

Although practically any area of the face can be augmented, there are a few considerations based on anatomic site. The nasojugal crease and temples are the sites most prone to postoperative "lumpiness" or

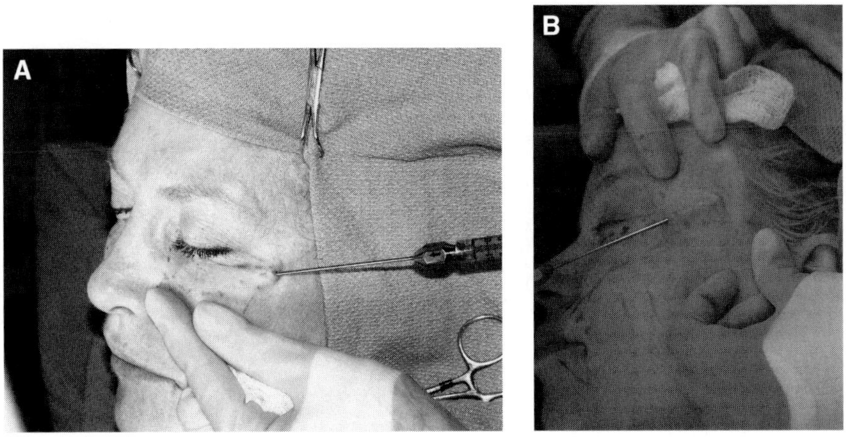

Fig. 6. (*A*, *B*) The zygomatic arch incision is used, through which most of the facial regions can be augmented.

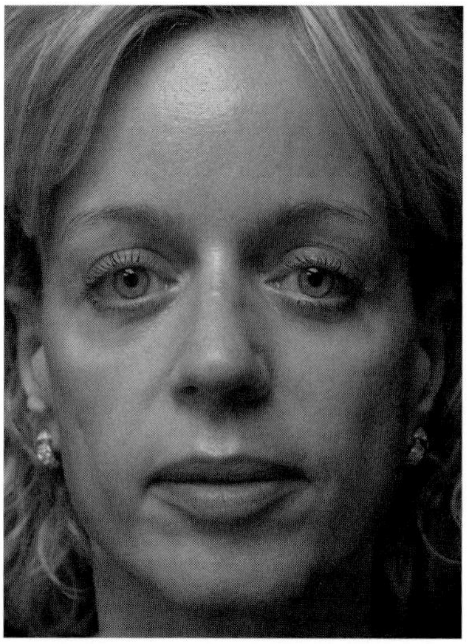

Fig. 8. Aging changes of the periorbital region accelerated by a prior transcutaneous lower blepharoplasty showing a visible infraorbital rim, a "tear-trough" deformity, and lateral canthal tendon laxity.

visible fat grafts. In contrast, the perioral region is the area most likely to lose a larger percentage of the grafted fat due to the high mobility of this area that comes with smiling, chewing, and talking.

Fat augmentation—anatomic considerations

Periorbital region

The aging changes of the periorbital region result in brow ptosis, dermatochalasis, hollowing of the infraorbital region, or pseudoherniation of the infraorbital fat pads (Fig. 8). Volume restoration of this region has the most profound and gratifying effects yet is the most challenging for a surgeon new to fat augmentation.

The importance of marking the patient in an upright position cannot be overemphasized. When the patient is recumbent, the area that needs to be augmented is obscured. The lateral zygomatic incision is used. A Coleman No. 2 cannula is advanced in a plane under the orbicularis oculi muscle, over the orbital septum, to reach the nasal sidewall. As the cannula is withdrawn, 0.05 mL of fat is placed in small parcels. Occasionally, it is necessary to start the injection at the nasal sidewall so that the fat will "fall" into place in the nasojugal crease when the cannula is withdrawn. Extreme care is taken to avoid overinjection of fat. Approximately 0.5 to 2 mL of fat are used for this area.

A lateral eyebrow incision (straight cannula) or the zygomatic incision (curved cannula) can be used to place fat into the brow region and the upper eyelid. Again, care is taken to not place too large a parcel of fat. The goal is to reproduce the natural fullness of a youthful brow and upper eyelid. Occasionally, this procedure may eliminate the need for an upper-eyelid blepharoplasty or a brow-lift if the redundant skin is addressed with volume restoration.

Cheeks

The malar region is also addressed from the zygomatic incision. After addressing the infraorbital rim, the cannula is withdrawn almost completely and then redirected in a fanning pattern across the malar eminence (Fig. 9). The fat is infiltrated into three layers: subcutaneous, intramuscular, submuscular/supraperiosteal. Each new layer is entered by withdrawing the cannula almost completely and then redirecting it superficially or deeply into the desired tissue plane. Approximately 2 to 6 mL of fat are used per side.

The lateral cheeks are addressed only in a superficial and middle plane to avoid injury to the underlying parotid gland. Care is taken to ensure an even distribution of fat in the subcutaneous plane. In addition, it is prudent to not overfill this region so as to maintain a slight arch to the zygoma in relation to the cheek. Approximately 2 to 10 mL of fat are used per side.

The jawline is best addressed from the angle of the mandible, at the base of the ear lobe and from the zygomatic incision. In this region, fat is best placed along the periosteum and in the muscle and subcuta-

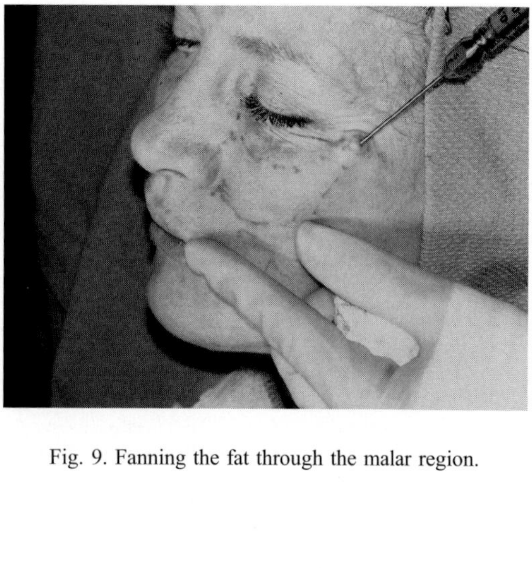

Fig. 9. Fanning the fat through the malar region.

neous planes. Care is taken to avoid trauma to the marginal mandibular nerve and the facial artery as they cross over the body of the mandible. Approximately 2 to 4 mL of fat are used per side.

Temples

Atrophy of the temples is particularly evident in thinner-faced individuals. Fat is infiltrated conservatively in this region due to the risk of contour irregularities. Either a zygomatic incision or a hairline incision can be used. The cannula is inserted in a plane running over the superficial temporoparietal fascia. Fat augmentation is performed in a radial pattern, with care not to overcorrect or create lumps. Approximately 2 to 4 mL of fat are used per side. Any irregularities are smoothed out with manual pressure.

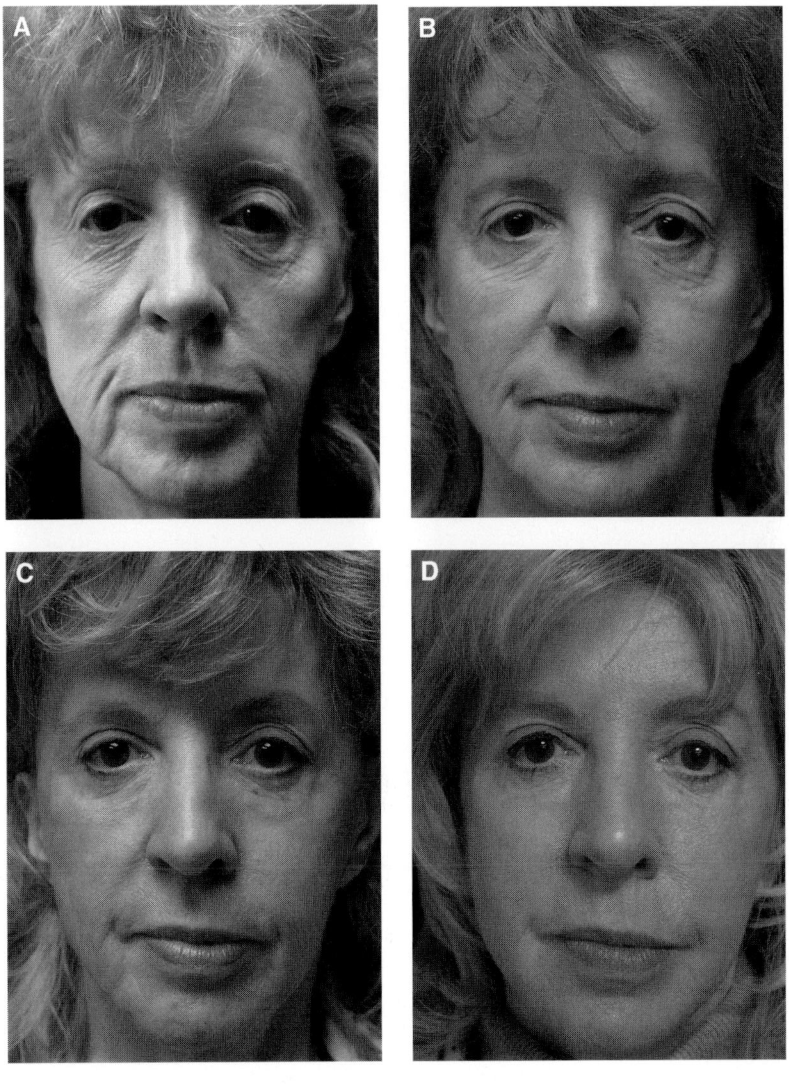

Fig. 10. (*A*) A 65-year-old woman who is 4 years out from a face-lift, lower eye-lift, and cheek implants now showing significant volume loss/skeletonization, lateral canthal tendon laxity, and visible cheek implants. (*B*) One year after first session of autologous fat augmentation of the midface/perioral region. (*C*) Eight months after second session of autologous fat augmentation, cantopexy, and and Obagi Blue-Peel for periorbital rhytides. (*D*) Four months after third session of autologous fat augmentation. In this photograph, the patient is 2 years older than in (*A*).

Repeat procedures

Patients with thinner faces may require more than one fat grafting session. Patients are informed that they may require one to three procedures to achieve the desired result. Usually, the final result is evident by 3 months. Therefore, sessions are spaced no sooner than 3 months apart so that the final result of each session is appreciated before the addition of more fat. Figs. 10 through 13 show typical before and after results for patients across a wide age range.

Complications

Infection

Particular care should be taken to ensure sterility during the entire harvesting, preparation, and infiltration of the fat to minimize the risks of infection. In over 200 cases, the author has encountered only one infection, which responded appropriately to systemic antibiotics. The author does not routinely prescribe prophylactic antibiotics. The literature supports the

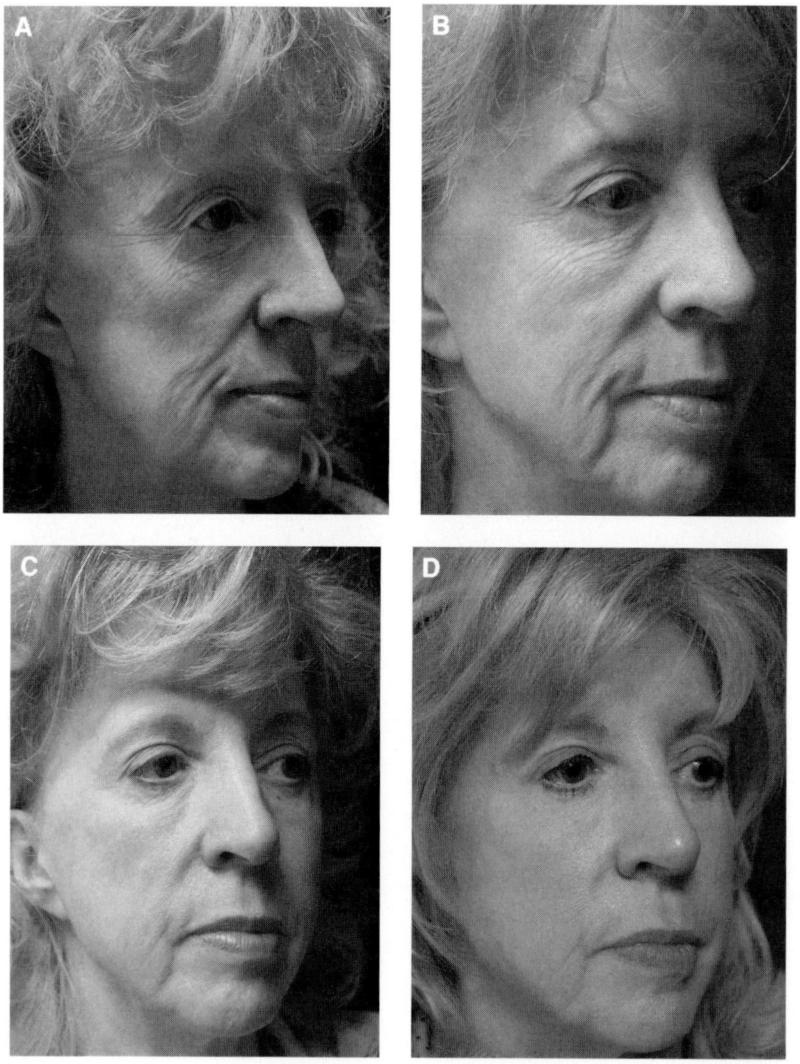

Fig. 11. Oblique views of patient in Fig. 11 showing the lifting of the excess skin of the cheeks by fat augmentation. (*A*) Preoperative. (*B*) One year after first session. (*C*) Eight months after second session. (*D*) Four months after third fat transfer.

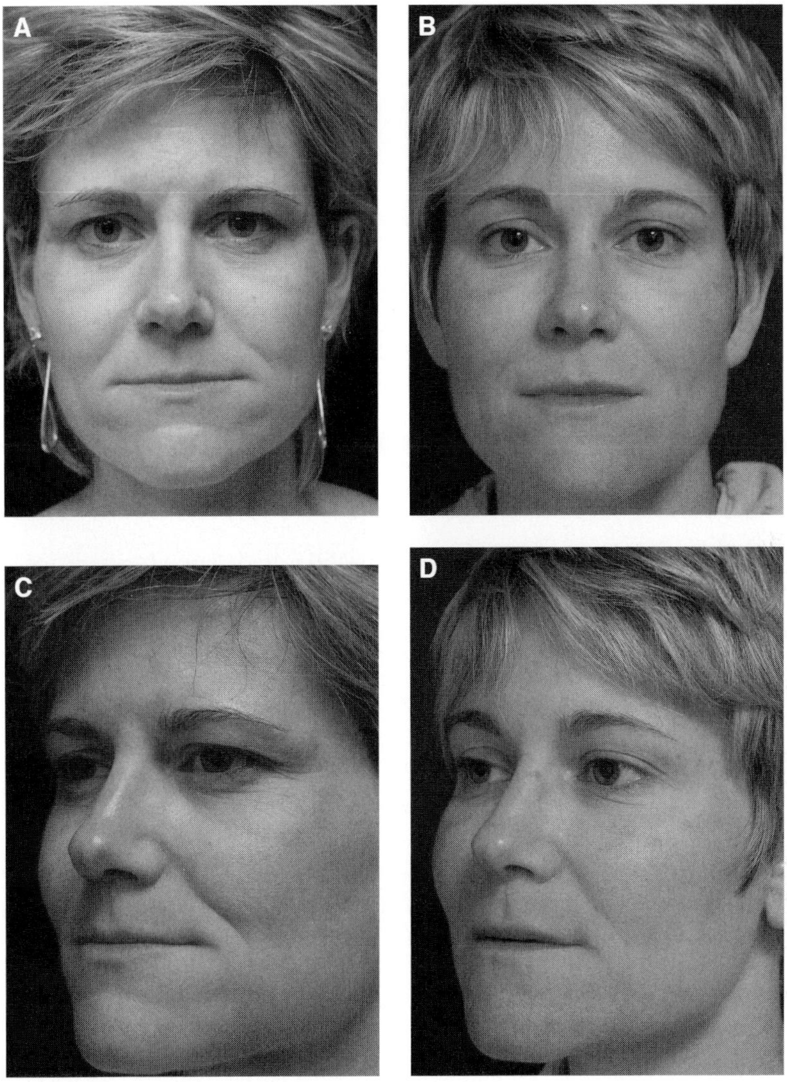

Fig. 12. (*A*) A young female patient with a square face, brow ptosis, and infraorbital hollowing. (*B*) Fourteen months after endoscopic brow-lift and 9 months after second autologous fat transfer showing a more rounded cheek, improved infraorbital hollowing, softened nasolabial folds, and an overall more feminine appearance. (*C*) Preoperative oblique view. (*D*) Postoperative oblique view.

low incidence of infection in fat augmentation patients; however, there is a report of a patient developing an infection with *Mycobacteria xenopi* from a possible dental abscess [17]. To further minimize the risk of infection, the surgeon must be cognizant of any additional procedures the patient may have had in the few weeks leading up to surgery. The author reported on a case of dacryocystitis that followed the placement of punctal plugs in a patient with an undiagnosed lacrimal duct obstruction [18]. The timing of the plug placement and the development of the infection occurred 3 days after the fat augmentation surgery, thus making the diagnosis of dacryocystitis more difficult. The patient did well after appropriate antibiotics and two dacryocystorhinostomy surgeries.

Extreme care should be taken to minimize perforation of the oral mucosa when placing fat in a deep plane. If perforation should occur, then the instrument responsible should be removed from the sterile field

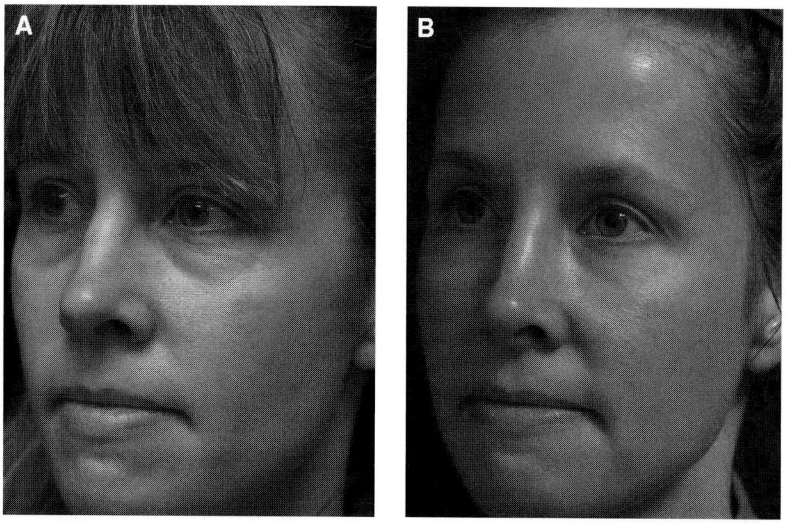

Fig. 13. (*A*) Infraorbital hollowing with malar atrophy. (*B*) Fifteen months after autologous fat augmentation.

and appropriate antibiotics that would cover oral flora started. The perioral region and lips are usually augmented last to prevent any inadvertent spread bacteria from an unsuspected mucosal perforation.

Embolization

There have been several reports in the literature of fat embolization secondary to inadvertent intravascular injection of the fat [19,20]. Most cases involved the use of sharp needles or syringes that were larger than 1 mL. The sharp needle can result in cannulation of a vessel while the large syringe can result in an injection of an inadvertent "bolus" of fat due to the increased force required to inject fat when using a 3- to 10-mL syringe. The author recommends only using blunt instruments for the placement of fat into any plane of the face, with the exception of the subdermal plane in which there is an absence of larger vessels. A further safeguard against intravascular injections includes the use of epinephrine in the nerve blocks and in the local anesthetic to promote vasoconstriction.

Weight loss/weight gain

Patients who wish to lose weight are encouraged to do so before fat augmentation. The author has had several patients who initially showed very good results but lost the volume by subsequent dieting. Alternately, moderate weight gain can result in hypertrophy of the grafted fat [21,22]. The hypertrophy may be enough that intervention is required in the form of dieting, liposuction, or direct surgical excision.

Cryopreservation

It is controversial to what extent frozen fat maintains viable adipocytes. Although freezing fat can diminish the number of viable adipocytes, there are some remaining cells that can survive and grow [23–26]. Any residual harvested fat is labeled with the patient's name and frozen for up to 1 year at −20°C. Frozen fat is used for small touch-ups in a fashion similar to how one would use other soft tissue fillers such as collagen or hyaluronic acid. If the patient requires a significant amount of volume augmentation, then only fresh fat is used.

Future considerations

Although fat transfers in various forms have been performed for over a century, the body of scientific knowledge in this field is growing rapidly. The future of fat augmentation is exciting as we begin to elucidate ways of improving fat graft survival. Furthermore, the field of stem cell research may help direct us in the proper placement of the grafts to better replicate the structure we wish to augment (muscle, fat, bone). We may find ourselves one day only injecting stem cells (preadipocytes) rather than the larger fat grafts. Our patients will be grateful to regain their natural look of youth without the appearance of having surgery.

References

[1] Hamra ST. A study of the long-term effect of malar fat repositioning in face lift surgery: short-term success but long-term failure. Plast Reconstr Surg 2002;110(3): 940–51 [discussion: 952–9].

[2] Pessa JE, Zadoo VP, Mutimer KL, et al. Relative maxillary retrusion as a natural consequence of aging: combining skeletal and soft-tissue changes into an integrated model of midfacial aging. Plast Reconstr Surg 1998;102(1):205–12.

[3] Gosain AK, Amarante MTJ, Hyde JS, et al. A dynamic analysis of changes in the nasolabial fold using magnetic resonance imaging: implications for facial rejuvenation and facial animation surgery. Plast Reconstr Surg 1996;98(4):622–36.

[4] Donofrio LM. Fat distribution: a morphologic study of the aging face. Dermatol Surg 2000;26(12): 1107–12.

[5] Coleman SR. Concepts of aging: rethinking the obvious. In: Coleman S, editor. Structural fat grafting. St. Louis (MO): Quality Medical Publishing; 2004. p. xvii–xxiv.

[6] Rohrich RJ, Sorokin ES, Brown SA. In search of improved fat transfer viability: a quantitative analysis of the role of centrifugation and harvest site. Plast Reconstr Surg 2004;113(1):391–5 [discussion: 396–7].

[7] Moore Jr JH, Kolaczynski JW, Morales LM, et al. Viability of fat obtained by syringe suction lipectomy: effects of local anesthesia with lidocaine. Aesthetic Plast Surg 1995;19(4):335–9.

[8] Shiffman MA, Kaminski MV. Fat transfer to the face: technique and new concepts. Facial Plast Surg Clin N Am 2001;9(2):229–37, viii.

[9] Smith J, Kaminski Jr MV, Wolosewick J. Use of human serum albumin to improve retention of autologous fat transplant. Plast Reconstr Surg 2002;109(2): 814–6.

[10] Rose JG, Lucarelli MJ, Lemke BN, et al. Histologic comparison of autologous fat processing methods. Ophthalmic Plastic and Reconstructive Surgery, In press.

[11] Rieck B, Schlaak S. Measurement in vivo of the survival rate in autologous adipocyte transplantation. Plast Reconstr Surg 2003;111(7):2315–23.

[12] Guerrerosantos J, Gonzalez-Mendoza A, Masmela Y, et al. Long-term survival of free fat grafts in muscle: an experimental study in rats. Aesthetic Plast Surg 1996;20(5):403–8.

[13] Butterwick KJ, Lack EA. Facial volume restoration with the fat autograft muscle injection technique. Dermatol Surg 2003;29(10):1019–26.

[14] Amar RE. Fat autograft muscle injections. Presented at the Annual Meeting of the American Academy of Cosmetic Surgery (AACS). Hollywood, Florida. February 2004.

[15] Rieck B, Schlaak S. In vivo tracking of rat preadipocytes after autologous transplantation. Ann Plast Surg 2003;51(3):294–300.

[16] Carraway JH, Mellow CG. Syringe aspiration and fat concentration: a simple technique for autologous fat injection. Ann Plast Surg 1990;24(3):293–6 [discussion: 297].

[17] Berman M. Rejuvenation of the upper eyelid complex with autologous fat transplantation. Dermatol Surg 2000;26(12):1113–6.

[18] Obagi S. Autologous fat augmentation and periorbital laser resurfacing complicated by abscess formation. Am J Cosmet Surg 2003;20(3):155–7.

[19] Feinendegen DL, Baumgartner RW, Vuadens P, et al. Autologous fat injection for soft tissue augmentation in the face: a safe procedure? Aesthetic Plast Surg 1998;22(3):163–7.

[20] Yoon SS, Chang DI, Chung KC. Acute fatal stroke immediately following autologous fat injection into the face. Neurology 2003;61(8):1151–2.

[21] Niechajev I, Sevcuk O. Long-term results of fat transplantation: clinical and histologic studies. Plast Reconstr Surg 1994;94(3):496–506.

[22] Miller JJ, Popp JC. Fat hypertrophy after autologous fat transfer. Ophthalmic Plast Reconstr Surg 2002; 18(3):228–31.

[23] Bertossi D, Kharouf S, d'Agostino A, et al. Facial localized cosmetic filling by multiple injections of fat stored at -30 degrees C. Techniques, clinical follow-up of 99 patients and histological examination of 10 patients. Ann Chir Plast Esthet 2000;45(5):548–55 [discussion: 555–6].

[24] Ullmann Y, Shoshani O, Fodor L, et al. Long-term fat preservation. J Drugs Dermatol 2004;3(3):266–9.

[25] Shoshani O, Ullmann Y, Shupak A, et al. The role of frozen storage in preserving adipose tissue obtained by suction-assisted lipectomy for repeated fat injection procedures. Dermatol Surg 2001;27(7): 645–7.

[26] Lidagoster MI, Cinelli PB, Levee EM, et al. Comparison of autologous fat transfer in fresh, refrigerated, and frozen specimens: an animal model. Ann Plast Surg 2000;44(5):512–5.

ELSEVIER
SAUNDERS

Oral Maxillofacial Surg Clin N Am 17 (2005) 111 – 121

ORAL AND MAXILLOFACIAL SURGERY CLINICS of North America

Minimally Invasive Face-lifting: S-Lift and S-Plus Lift Rhytidectomies

Steven B. Hopping, MD, FACS

The Center for Cosmetic Surgery, 2240 M Street NW, Suite 205, Washington, DC 20037-1404, USA

Today, many patients seeking facial rejuvenation desire a more limited procedure devoid of complications, with a natural, "nonplasticized" look and a rapid return to their usual activities. Patients often demonstrate their aesthetic desires for rejuvenation by lifting the skin of their faces with their fingers from the angle of the mandible vertically upward toward the crown of the head. This maneuver is one they have repeated endless times in the mirror before presenting for consultation (Fig. 1). It is important to remember that there is no surgical procedure more elective than face-lift surgery. Consequently, cosmetic surgeons must continually strive to maximize results while minimizing complications and postoperative recovery. Patients' wishes, as outlined earlier, may not always be shared by all cosmetic surgeons, many of whom often prefer a more aggressive surgical facial rejuvenation program. Recent reports of serious sequelae or even death associated with face-lift surgeries have patients questioning the value of aggressive face-lifts and lengthy anesthesia [1]. Sam Hamra [2] eloquently described the highly sophisticated, and technically challenging composite rhytidectomy in 1993, completing a trend toward more aggressive, lengthier multiplanar procedures. Perhaps not surprising, a concomitant increase in facial nerve injuries and dyskinesias was noted, precipitating Seckel's [3] 1994 publication, "Facial Danger Zones. Avoiding Nerve Injury in Facial Plastic Surgery." Seckel, a neurologist and a plastic surgeon, is a particular expert on facial nerve injuries. He noted in the preface of his book that he was referred three face-lift–related facial nerve injuries in 1 month, two following "composite" face-lifting. Seckel [3] further stated

> With today's more aggressive and deeper facial dissection in the course of the face-lift surgery, the peripheral nerves of the face are more often exposed, lie closer to the plane of dissection, and in my opinion are more likely to be injured. Injury to one of the major jacial nerve branches creates a catastrophe and occasionally irreversible facial deformity. Even patients who do recover muscle function following injury are often left with permanent involuntary muscle twitching or distortion of the facies by contracture and shortening of partially denervated muscles. Additionally, interruption of one of the major sensory nerves in the face can result in permanent disability secondary to numbness or, worse, intractable dysesthesia and pain.

In the author's opinion, with the timing of Seckel's book, the swing of the pendulum toward more aggressive face-lifting reached it pinnacle. Enter the S-Lift, a short-scar, "short-flap" face-lift technique reintroduced by Saylan in 1999 [4]. Previously, Skoog [5] revolutionized rhytidectomy by describing the importance of submuscular aponeurotic system

E-mail address: steven@stevenbhopping.md

1042-3699/05/$ – see front matter
doi:10.1016/j.coms.2004.09.006

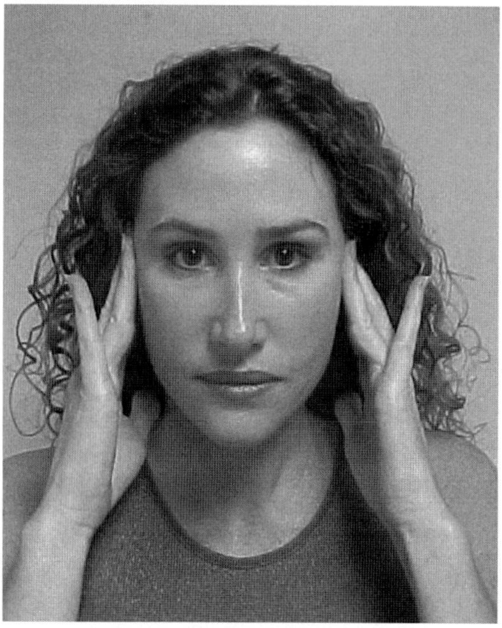

Fig. 1. Patient demonstrating the results she would like to achieve from face-lifting. Note the primarily vertical vector of this mock rejuvenation.

(SMAS) lifting. The S-Lift combined the advantages of a limited incision and dissection with the advantages of SMAS lifting and manipulation. Saylan's original contribution to the technique involved the effective use of purse-string sutures suspending the moblie SMAS and the extended SMAS platysma (ESP) to the fixed periosteum-facia of the zygomatic arch [4]. In the properly selected patient, the S-Lift can achieve much of our patients' "wish list" for facial rejuvenation—providing natural aesthetic improvement in a limited operation with minimal risks and a short recovery period. The purpose of this article is to describe the principles of this short-scar approach (the S-Lift) and to describe an advanced variation of the technique designed to improve midfacial aging (the S-Plus Lift).

The S-Lift is a conceptually new approach to face-lifting and is particularly applicable to younger patients and patients requiring secondary face-lifts. It is important to note that the S-Lift is not a simple "minilift" skin excision but an advanced SMAS multiplane rhytidectomy. In this article, the author also describes what is referred to as the "S-Plus Lift." This procedure combines aspects of the technique of lateral SMASectomy described by Baker [6] and malar fat pad suspension using a purse-string suture, suspending the ptotic malar fat pad from the temporalis fascia (M suture) described by Tonnard et al [7]. The S-Plus Lift extends the efficacy of S-Lift in those patients who have significant midfacial ptosis. The S-Lift is generally a short-flap face-lift procedure, whereas the S-Plus with its midface extension, is a "long-flap" rhytidectomy.

Advantages of the S-Lift

Limited incisions and scars

Limited incisions translates clinically to limited scarring. The S-Lift provides full access to the midface, jawline, and neck through an incision that is principally limited to the preauricular area. Accessibility can further be enhanced by extending the incision into the temporal scalp with a pretrichael or C-shaped vertical limb. This extension allows a more complete subcutaneous dissection in the temple that can be extended to the malar eminence and orbicularis complex. This extension is particularly helpful in performing the SMASectomy resection and advancement in the midface and for placing the M suture from the temporalis fascia to the malar fat pad complex. The S-Lift avoids a lengthy scar in the postauricular hairline and can be considered "ponytail friendly."

Minimized risk

The limited-incision design of the S-Lift precludes extensive dissection in the posterior–inferior neck, minimizing risk to the most commonly injured nerve in face-lifting: the great auricular nerve. There is also a rich vascular supply in the posterior–inferior neck region; avoiding sharp dissection in the region reduces the likelihood of bruising and hematoma.

Primarily vertical vector rejuvenation

A key component to a successful aesthetic outcome is the principally vertical rotation of the cheek/neck flap. This rotation gives significant improvement in the cheek, jowl, and neckline without the "windsweep," pulled look of a more posterior vector lift. This vertical rotation is perpendicular to the myelolabial fold and opposes the downward gravitational pull on the facial tissues.

Excellent neck and jowl rejuvenation

The "O" and "U" purse-string SMAS plication sutures allow excellent "block and tackle" lifting of these structures. The more mobile SMAS and ESP are maneuvered vertically by the purse-string sutures to the rigidly fixed periosteum and ligamentous structures of the zygomatic arch.

Reduced surgical and anesthesia time

Although speed is not necessarily a priority in cosmetic surgery, it is a known surgical adage that shorter anesthesia times are associated with fewer complications. Reducing the time on the face-lift closure allows the surgeon the luxury of adding some accessory procedures that often enhance the aesthetic outcome. These might include minimal-incision brow-lift, midline platysmaplasty, midface lift, buccal fat reduction, or cheek and chin augmentation with implants to allow a truly three-dimensional rejuvenation.

SMAS procedure

The S-Lift is not just a "skin" lift but advances and tightens the SMAS network of facial support. The U and O and M sutures are SMAS plication sutures. The SMASectomy resection and repair is a true SMAS imbrication. Indeed, even a "deep plane" lift through a limited S-Lift incision can be accomplished. The possibilities are limited only by the imagination.

Short recovery period

The generally shorter-flap S-Lift is associated with less bruising, less edema, and faster recovery of the healing response. The more limited incision and dissection results in less surface area of healing. Shorter scars mean less crusting and less "wounding" response and collagen deposition. The absence of incisions in the postauricular scalp means less hair loss and less temporary and permanent alopecia.

Disadvantages of the S-Lift

Limited access to the neck

Surgical exposure to the neck is somewhat compromised in limited-incision procedures such as the S-Lift compared with the more classical rhytidectomy approach. The novice surgeon may particularly be bothered by this limited exposure and the resultant difficulty with instrumentation. Visualization of the neck can significantly be improved by extending the S-Lift incision 1 to 2 cm postauricularly. This maneuver allows markedly improved visualization of the posterior, inferior, and anterior neck structures including the sternocleidomastoid muscle, angle of the mandible, and the ESP for ease of placement of the O suture.

Posterior "dog ear" that can last 1 to 3 months and require revision surgery

There are a number of tricks to help avoid this postoperative sequela, including wide undermining of the short postauricular limb of the incision, liposculpture of the posterior neck from this incision, and initiating closure from posterior to anterior using the technique of "halfing" the unequaled flap with interrupted mattress sutures that also pick up fascia in the area.

Pain over the zygomatic arch secondary to the O and U suture

This complication usually is temporary and self-limiting. Triamcinolone (Kenalog) injections (5 to 10 mg per cc) have been beneficial in speeding the resolution of this problem. Ultimately, the suture can be removed under local anesthesia if symptoms persist.

Palpability of "knot" of the U and O suture

Again, suture removal can be performed in obvious cases. The author has changed from using permanent 2-0 Ethibond suture (Ethicon) to dissolvable 2-0 Vicryl (Ethicon).

Extrusion of the U and O suture through the skin

This problem can be avoided by "burying" the knot of the suture with a dissolvable suture. In extremely thin-skinned patients, the O and U suture should be avoided or a dissolvable suture placed such as 2-0 Vicryl.

Limited improvement on severely ptotic or aged necks

Many of these cases can markedly be improved by combining S-Lift with midline platysmaplasty.

Some cases are simply best served by extending to a postauricular incision with the additional vector of pull and skin excision.

Limited improvement in patients with ptotic midface

These patients need the S-Plus Lift, with extension well into the midface, or SMASectomy or M suture suspension of the malar fat. Subperiosteal midface lift and cheek implants also are possibilities for these patients.

Key technical points

- Use retrotragal incision in men and women, except for smokers in whom a pretragal incision is recommended (Fig. 2).
- Pre-excision of a limited skin ellipse should be conservative; skin only; stay superficial. Pre-excision is less important for pretragal incisions.
- Use a No. 15 blade to create thick flaps and demarcate the dissection plane just superficial to the parotid fascia; use the blade in a " bevel up" fashion.
- Complete flap elevation under direct vision with face-lift scissors. Direct visualization is particularly important in revision rhytidectomy in which normal tissue planes may have been disrupted.
- The extent of undermining is determined by extent of midface laxity (the greater the midfacial laxity, the greater the undermining).
- Perform closed and open liposuction only after elevation of flap to maximize flap viability.
- Identify the ESP. Grasp the ESP with a long forceps and evaluate the ideal location for elevation and rotation with the U suture.
- Place U suture (2-0 Vicryl) from the zygomatic arch vertically inferior to a point approximately 1 to 2 cm inferior and posterior to the angle of the mandible (Fig. 3).
- Placement of O suture (2-0 Vicryl) is again from the zygomatic arch toward the jowl to tighten the jowl and achieve some midface tightening (see Fig. 3).
- Use an M suture (4-0 Vicryl) for midface lifting from the temporalis fascia to the malar fat pad (purse-string suture) (see Fig. 3).
- SMASectomy resection and plication is ideal to enhance midface elevation in patients with excessive midface ptosis (Fig. 4).
- Use a flap demarcator to accurately measure the amount of skin that can safely be excised (Fig. 5).
- Check for complete hemostasis. A "second look" technique is recommended before closure. (Complete the dissection on the right side apply temporary fixation sutures or surgical clips, do the same on the left side, return to the right side to recheck hemostasis and close.)
- Perform flap rotation to achieve a primarily vertical vector lift. This vector of rotation is key to achieve the optimal results and avoid the "wind tunnel" look.
- The initial key closure is C-to-C_1, followed by A-to-A_1 and B-to-B_1. Point C is under the most tension; no tension on points A or B (Fig. 6).
- Sew flap (C-to-C_1) firmly to temporalis fascia with horizontal mattress suture of 3-0 Vicryl at point C.
- Close the posterior and temple dog-ear redundancies first.
- The S-design horizontal temporal incision and excision preserves the temporal hairline while removing the temporal dog ear (Fig. 7).
- Two-layer closure (4-0 Vicryl in subcutaneous layer and 5-0 fast-absorbing plain or intracuticular or 5-0 Monocryl (Ethicon) for the skin) provides the final closure (Fig. 8).
- Perform autogenous fat grafting to smile, frown, and marionette lines and lips. Part of aging is gravity, but a large part of aging is atrophy. Effective rejuvenation must lift and fill.

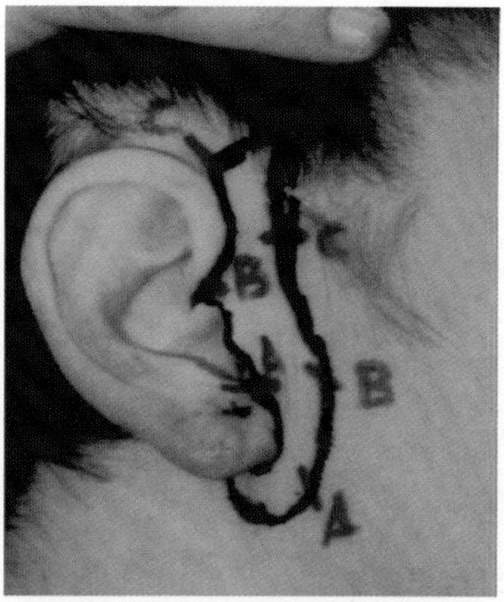

Fig. 2. S-Lift incision demonstrating three key vectors: A to A_1, B to B_1, and C to C_1.

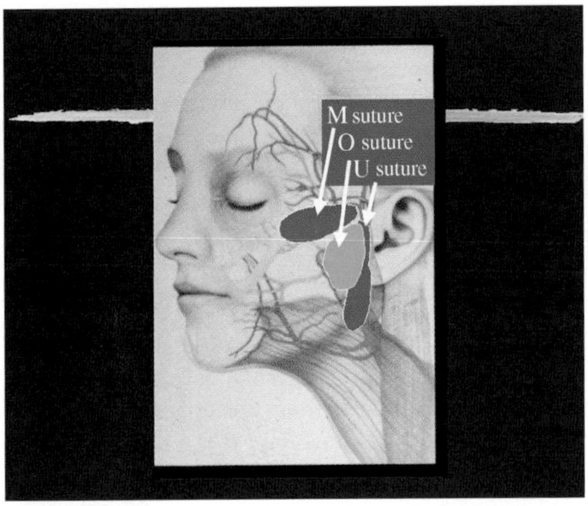

Fig. 3. Diagramatic depiction of U suture, O suture, and M suture.

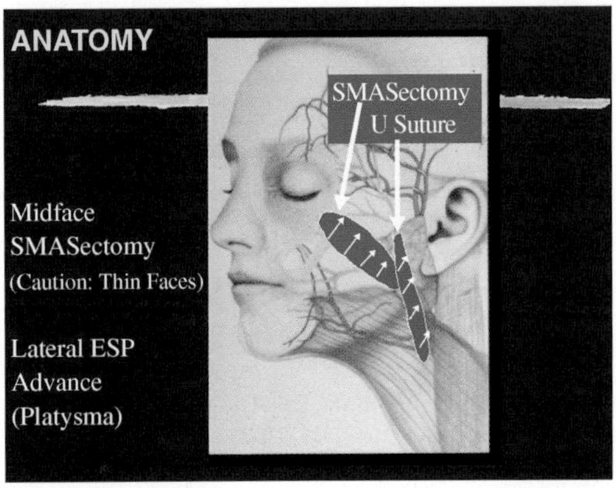

Fig. 4. S-Plus Lift with planned U suture and SMASectomy outlined.

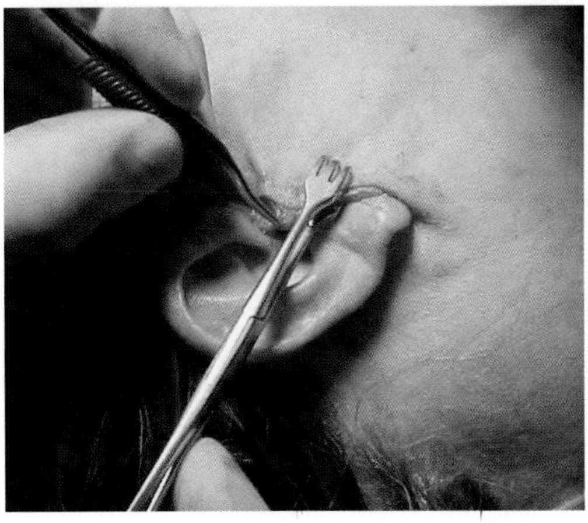

Fig. 5. Flap demarcator is used for precise measurement of flap excision.

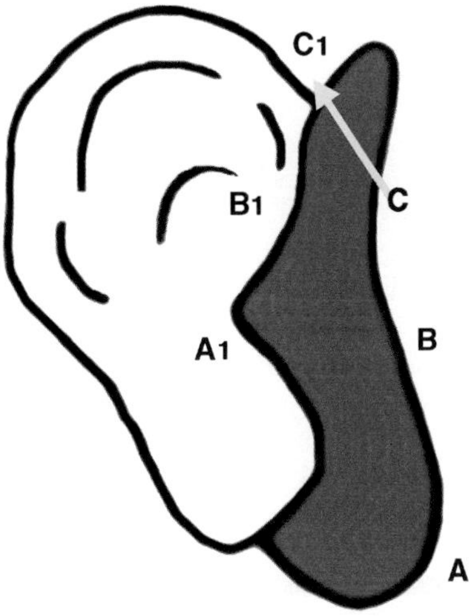

Fig. 6. The initial key suture is placed by advancing C-to-C_1 in a primarily vertical vector.

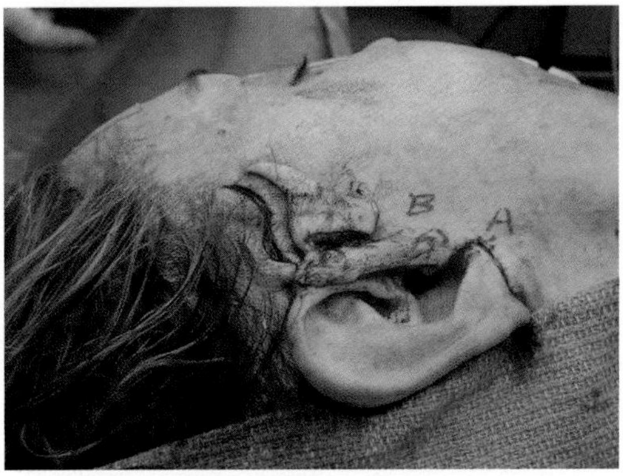

Fig. 7. A horizontal S-incision preserves the temporal hair tuft while correcting the superior "dog ear."

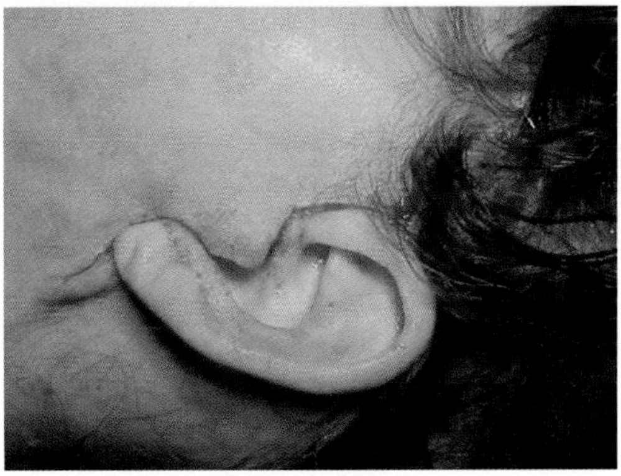

Fig. 8. Final closure. Note the skin redundancy over the tragus to prevent tragal contracture and deformity.

Indications

S-Lift (short flap) is indicated in patients who have mild-to-moderate neck laxity, without platysma banding at rest, and mild-to-moderate jowl laxity. Often, the S-Lift will also require neck and jowl liposuction or chin augmentation or both (Table 1, Figs. 9, 10, and 13).

S-Plus Lift (long flap) with midface extension is indicated in patients who have moderate-to-severe midface laxity/ptosis and malar insufficiency. The M suture or SMASectomy gives midface elevation and rejuvenation (Table 1, Figs. 11 and 14).

S-Lift or S-Plus Lift with platysmaplasty is indicated in patients who have platysma banding at rest (Table 1, Fig. 15).

Table 1
Clinical indications for S-Lift rhytidectomy

Clinical findings	Procedure
Mild-to-moderate neck laxity, mild-to-moderate jowling	S-Lift (short flap)
Moderate-to-severe neck laxity, moderate-to-severe jowling, midfacial laxity	S-Plus Lift (long flap)
Platysma banding at rest	S-Lift, S-Plus Lift with midline platysmaplasty

A retrospective review of 200 consecutive cases

A retrospective review of 200 consecutive S-Lift and S-Plus Lift rhytidectomies performed from December 2001 to December 2003 was undertaken. All procedures were performed in a private AAAC-accredited cosmetic surgical office operating suite on patients under intravenous sedation anesthesia. Modified tumescent anesthesia was used (1000 mg normal saline mixed with 50 mg 1% xylocaine plain and 2 mg epinephrine). The satisfaction index of these patients was tabulated from postoperative questionnaires evaluated at 6 months (Fig. 12). Fifty-eight percent indicated that they were "very satisfied" with the results. Thirty-six percent were "satisfied," giving an overall satisfaction rate of 94%. Six percent of patients indicated that they were "not satisfied" with their aesthetic results. Patients not satisfied with the results at 6 or 12 months were offered secondary surgeries, which in most cases involved a secondary S-Lift, with or without a posterior limb. Such a secondary enhancement can readily be performed in 90 minutes. Comparatively, the author's revision rate for standard rhytidectomy is similar (5% to 7%).

A retrospective review of complications from these 200 cases revealed major hematoma in 4 cases (2%). These cases were S-Lift procedures and required return to the operating room, with opening of the flaps, control of bleeding, and drainage. Four cases (2%) of facial nerve palsies (2 of the buccal and

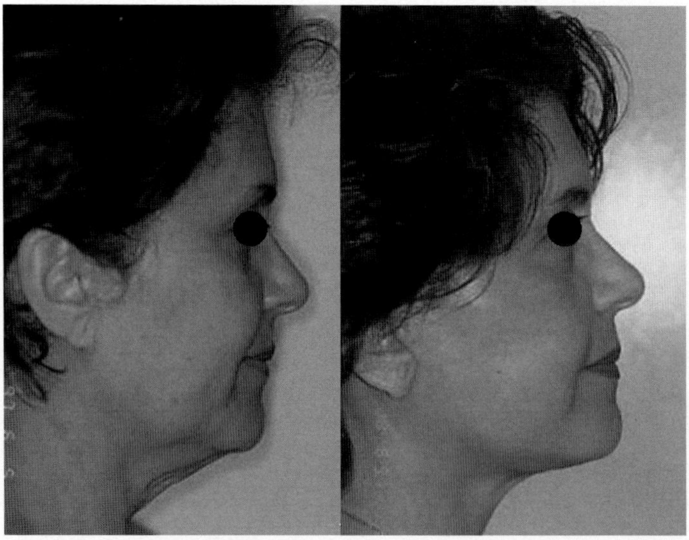

Fig. 9. S-Lift. Before and after six months. Note improved contour of neck and jowl line.

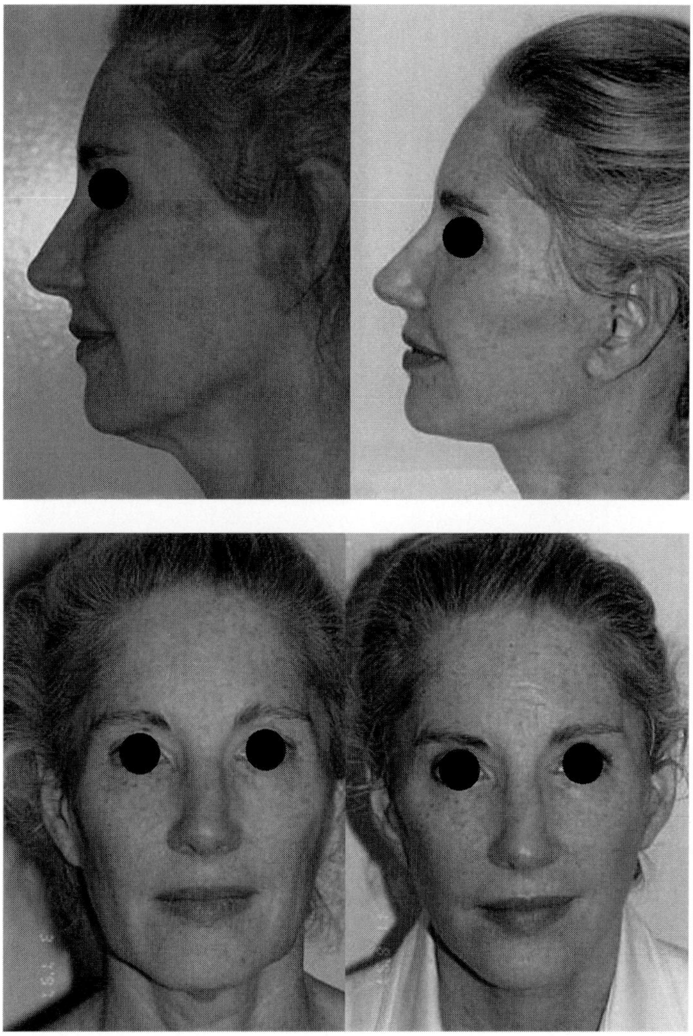

Fig. 10. S-Lift. Before and after. Note improvement in neck and jowl with preservation of temporal hair. Natural looking results.

2 of the ramis mandibularis branches) were noted. Each resolved with expectant treatment within 3 months. Two cases (1%) of parotid fistula were noted, which resolved with drainage and pressure dressings after 3 weeks. There was persistent pain over the zygomatic arch in four patients (2%), related to the U and O sutures, which resolved with dilute Kenalog injections (5 mg/ml) and time. There were 6 cases (3%) of hypertrophic preauricular scarring, treated with intralesional Kenalog (5 mg/ml) injections. There were 10 cases with unsatisfactory results (5%), requiring secondary surgeries. Six of these

Box 1. Complications in 200 consecutive S-Lift, S-Plus Lift patients

- Major hematoma (2%)
- Facial nerve palsies (temporary) (2%)
- Parotid fistula (1%)
- Persistent pain at zygomatic arch (2%)
- Hypertrophic preauricular scarring (3%)
- Infection (2%)
- Unsatisfactory aesthetic results (5%)

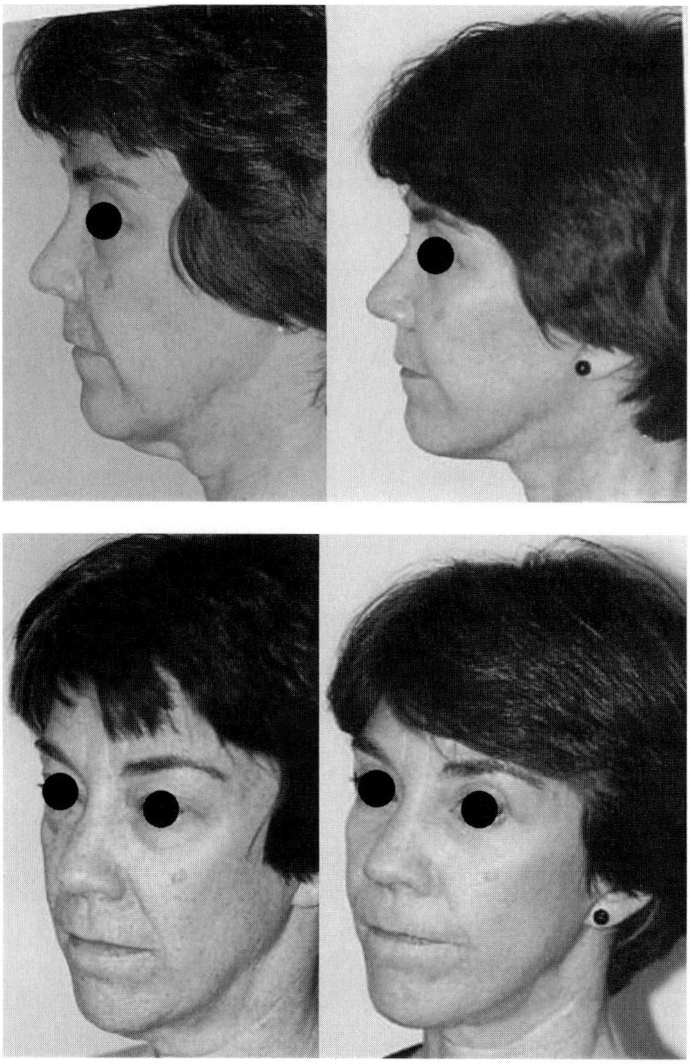

Fig. 11. S-Plus Lift. Before and after six months. Note midface elevation and more youthful cheek contour with SMASectomy and M-suture.

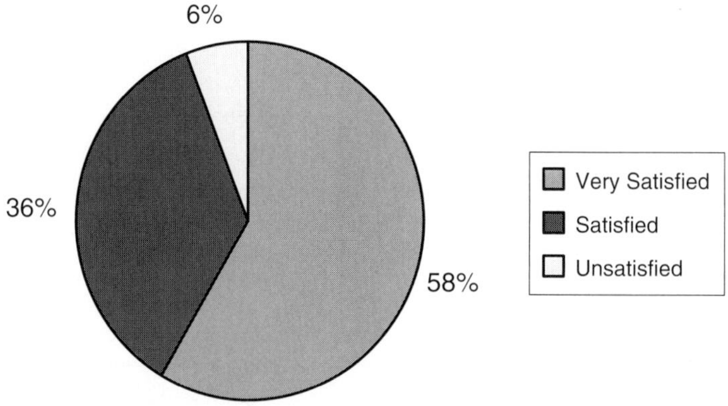

Fig. 12. Patient satisfaction survey at six months (200 consecutive S-Lifts, S-Plus Lifts).

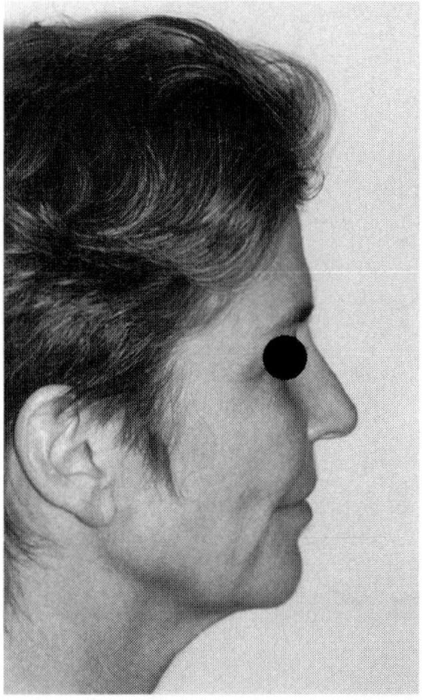

Fig. 13. Mild to moderate neck laxity, mild to moderate jowling. Excellent candidate for S-Lift.

were due to concern with earlobe redundancy or irregularities, necessitating a posterior flap. There were 4 cases of infection (2%) (Box 1).

Discussion

Following Hamra's [2] publication of composite rhytidectomy in 1992, the sophistication and technical challenge of face-lift surgery rose significantly. This trend was followed by an increase in serious postoperative sequelae including temporary and permanent dyskinesias and facial nerve injuries. As mentioned earlier, face-lifting is perhaps the most elective of all surgical procedures. Patients do not anticipate and, even if warned, do not accept long-term recovery or permanent adverse sequelae following face-lift surgery. Today, most patients, regardless of informed consent, expect an excellent aesthetic result without complications and with a rapid return to normal activities.

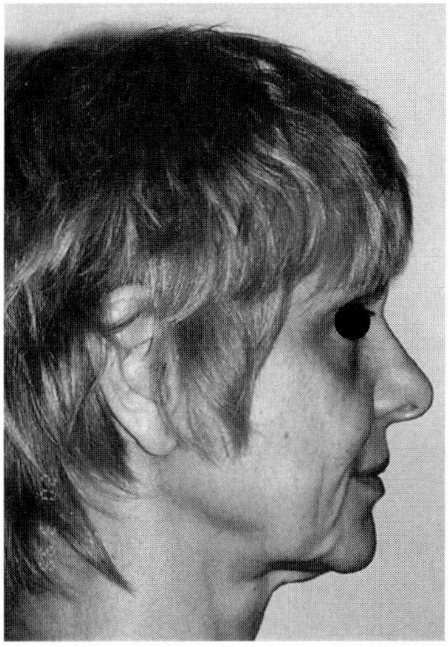

Fig. 14. Moderate neck laxity, moderate to severe jowling, mid facial laxity. Good indications for S-Plus Lift with SMASectomy or M-Suture to enhance the midface results.

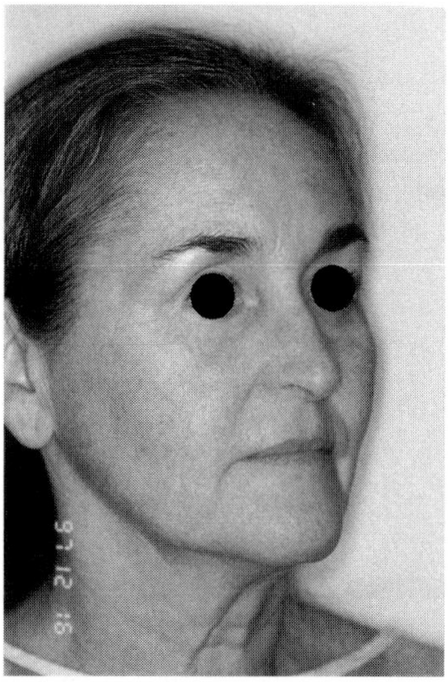

Fig. 15. Platysma banding at rest. This patient requires midline platysmaplasty.

The S-Lift and S-Plus Lift represent a return of the pendulum in the direction of less aggressive and less complicated rhytidectomy procedures. These procedures can provide the aesthetic results that patients desire while achieving their wishes for limited risks and an acceptably short recovery period. In the author's series, 94% of patients were either satisfied or very satisfied with their surgical outcomes. The most common problem with the procedure is inadequate correction in patients who have excess skin laxity or poor skin elasticity, necessitating a secondary "tuck-up" procedure at 6 to 12 months. This procedure is an easy one to offer patients and they readily accept a secondary procedure, particularly if their first experience was a positive one. Persistent earlobe redundancy or deformity is another cause for revision surgery.

The S-Lift and S-Plus Lift should not be construed as simple, skin-excision minilifts. They are complex face-lifts that incorporate SMAS lifting techniques and principles. Surgeons performing the S-Lift must possess an intimate knowledge of facial nerve anatomy, be able to control bleeding, and know how and when to convert to the more classical rhytidectomy techniques if necessary. In the author's series, hematomas, facial nerve palsies, parotid fistulas, hypertrophic scars, infections, and persistent neuralgias were encountered. The use of tumescent anesthesia and direct rather than blind dissection is strongly encouraged to preserve tissue planes and prevent facial nerve injuries. Direct visualization is particularly important for secondary rhytidectomies where tissue planes have been altered, making blind dissection particularly risky.

Not all patients are good candidates for S-Lift or S-Plus Lift and it behooves the cosmetic surgeon to select carefully patients who are well suited for this procedure. In the author's experience, this includes the younger patient who would like to be proactive in maintaining a youthful appearance, the patient who does not want an overpulled classical rhytidectomy stigmata, patients who have had previous face-lift surgery and now require a secondary procedure, and patients with a smoking history or who have medical problems dictating a short anesthetic and surgical procedure.

The S-Lift, as described by Saylan [4], is a short-flap SMAS face-lift that is safe, even in patients with a history of smoking, hypertension, controlled diabetes, or other medical problems. The vector of lift is vertical, which gives a natural appearance while providing rejuvenation to the neck and jowls. Careful attention must be given to creating and closing the temporal hair-sparing incision superiorly and the infralobular redundancy below the earlobe. The initial key suture is C-to-C$_1$, placed in a principally vertical rotation rather than A-to-A$_1$ as originally proposed by Saylan [4] (see Fig. 6).

The S-Plus Lift with midface extension using SMASectomy or malar fat pad suspension using the M suture is better suited for patients with moderate-to-severe midface laxity/ptosis (Fig. 14). The incision for the S-Lift and S-Plus Lift is exactly the same but the latter is a long-flap technique that requires dissection nearly to the myelolabial fold to perform the SMASectomy and malar fat pad elevation. The malar fat pad is not undermined but is suspended vertically from the temporalis fascia as a vascular pedicle using the purse-string M suture. S-Lift with or without midface extension combined with platysmaplasty is best for patients who demonstrate platysma bands at rest (see Fig. 15).

Summary

Rhytidectomy is perhaps the most elective of all surgical procedures. Over the past 2 decades, there has been a trend toward more technically challenging, multiplanar face-lift procedures requiring higher levels of technical expertise and longer operative and anesthesia times. Although difficult to document, there has been a suggestion of increased morbidity from these procedures. More important, there has been a rash of lay reports of complications and even deaths during cosmetic surgical procedures including face-lifting. Certainly, there are good indications for these more sophisticated procedures, especially for patients with advanced aging problems. Not every patient, however, should receive a deep plane or composite face-lift simply because they might be technically in vogue. Many patients now seeking facial rejuvenation simply do not require the aesthetic advantages that the more sophisticated face-lift procedures offer. Indeed, in many of these younger patients, such invasive procedures are contraindicated.

There is a definite paradigm shift in the expectations and motivations of today's well-informed face-lift patients. They are as concerned about the risks and the recovery from the procedures as they are about the aesthetic outcome. Few are willing to trade additional scarring or significantly lengthier recovery periods for a somewhat better, subjective aesthetic result. With all the information highlighting the few "tragedies" from cosmetic surgery, patients are indeed demanding safer and shorter procedures, less not more anesthesia, and more rapid return to normal activities. Despite the popularity of the television show "Extreme Makeovers," this concept is not what motivates most patients seeking facial rejuvenation. Most patients simply want to look their best and regain features that time has stolen from them. They do not want to look like someone else, and most do not want to look "operated." Much the way rhinoplasty aesthetics have become more conservative, with an attempt to preserve (not destroy) support structures, thereby achieving results that look less operated than their predecessors, face-lifting should be following a similar trend.

Procedures such as the S-Lift allow for less surgical and anesthetic time, leading to better outcomes for these elective outpatient cosmetic procedures. The efficiency of these operations also allows the bundling of procedures such as implants, browlift, facial rejuvenation with fat, and blepharoplasties that can enhance the overall aesthetic improvement without adding to morbidity or recovery.

Using the S-Lift and the S-Plus Lift for the indications previously outlined has resulted in a high overall patient satisfaction rate (94%) while achieving patients' desires for a limited procedure, minimal complications, natural-looking results, and a rapid return to normal activities.

References

[1] Green M, Adalo A. Dying to look good. People Magazine. March 22, 2004;89–93.
[2] Hamra S. Composite rhytidectomy. Plast Reconstr Surg J 1992;90:1–14.
[3] Seckel B. Facial danger zones. Avoiding injury in facial plastic surgery. St. Louis (MO): Quality Medical Publishing; 1994.
[4] Saylan Z. The S-Lift: less is more. Aesthetic Surg J 1999;19:406.
[5] Skoog T. Plastic surgery: new methods and refinements. Philadelphia: WB Saunders; 1974.
[6] Baker DC. Minimal incision rhytidectomy (short scar facelift) with lateral SMASectomy: evolution and application. Aesthet Surg J 2001;21:14.
[7] Tonnard P, Verpaele A, et al. Minimal access cranial suspension lift. A modified S-Lift. Plast Reconstr Surg J 2002;109:6.

ELSEVIER
SAUNDERS

Oral Maxillofacial Surg Clin N Am 17 (2005) 123 – 127

ORAL AND
MAXILLOFACIAL
SURGERY CLINICS
of North America

Legal Considerations Surrounding Cosmetic Surgery

W. Scott Johnson, Esquire

Hancock, Daniel, Johnson, and Nagle, PC, 4112 Innslake Drive, Glen Allen, VA 23060, USA

"Ms. Patient, I am attorney Johnson and I am here today to take your deposition in the medical malpractice case that you filed against your oral and maxillofacial surgeon. Please tell me what you recall about the day of surgery."

"I don't recall anything about the day that I had my face-lift, but I do remember word for word what I told my surgeon when I called him the day after I had my face-lift to report the swelling and the excruciating pain. . .."

As an oral and maxillofacial surgeon, you can take all of the appropriate steps and use all of the appropriate precautions, yet a medical malpractice claim against you will most often rise and fall on a single telephone call or office visit. Ask any plaintiff's attorney and you will hear that the overwhelming majority of patients who pursue medical malpractice cases do so because of lack of communication or poor communication by their health care provider. As an oral and maxillofacial surgeon, you may not be able to prevent complications from occurring but have significant control over enhancing quality communication with your patient.

This article presents practical views from the trenches on issues of past history, informed consent, preparation for a case, documentation, postoperative actions, and complications and addresses patient refunds and releases. With the demands on surgeons' schedules, I realize that asking a surgeon to talk more with a patient and document more in the patient's chart can be viewed as a bit of an oxymoron. Those surgeons who take the time to focus on detailed communications, however, will most often not find themselves embroiled in protracted litigation.

Past history

When a patient reports a history that includes the patient having received cosmetic treatment or having undergone cosmetic procedures at the hands of two other health care providers, an immediate alarm should sound in your mind. If two other providers rendered care to the patient and were unable to make the patient happy, do not let your ego convince you that you could be the first to succeed at this un-daunting challenge. Undoubtedly, residual problems continue to exist, making it difficult to establish the baseline from which you are starting.

It is not uncommon to learn from your patient history that the patient is taking sertraline hydrochloride (Zoloft) or other medication to allow them to cope with life or, as some patients phrase it, "to keep an even keel." It is prudent to explore in greater detail the status of a patient's emotional and mental well-being. If a patient has been taking 20 mg of Zoloft for 4 years without side effects, then additional investigation is probably not needed. If the patient has recently undergone significant mood swings or is experiencing significant increases or decreases in the dosing of medication, then it could impact his or her ability to withstand the procedure.

Each patient has different expectations. Some patients are realists and realize that cosmetic surgery will not fix all of their perceived deformities or problems but will give them the ability to turn back the clock on the natural aging process. Other individuals want to look perfect. Some have a movie-star

E-mail address: sjohnson@hdjn.com

doi:10.1016/j.coms.2004.10.006

mentality that is impossible to derail, and it is this group of patients that you should invite to seek further treatment elsewhere. Recommending that these patients seek a second opinion is a conservative approach to telling them that you are not comfortable proceeding with the surgery they have inquired about.

Significant past medical history that should not be overlooked are reports of anorexia, bulimia, or ongoing psychiatric therapy. The bottom line is to not operate within a vacuum. Make sure that the other treating health care providers know what the patient is seeking and what your treatment plan is going to be. A psychiatrist may realize that a patient seeking a cosmetic procedure is doing so as a defensive mechanism for some underlying mental illness and may be able to talk the patient out of it. Conferring with the family physician may lead to learning that the patient has been has been taking warfarin sodium (Coumadin) for 5 years but forgot to list it when identifying current medications.

Informed consent

Informed consent is probably one of the most discussed and dreaded legal requirements. Surgeons want patients to focus on a successful procedure, not the risks, benefits, and alternatives, some of which can include death.

Patients seem to learn better through the use of visual aids. It frequently is the case for patients to be given a Krames pamphlet when a patient undergoes a routine oral and maxillofacial surgery procedure such as an extraction of a third molar or an apicoectomy. As cosmetic surgery continues to become a prevalent area of practice for health care providers, it is anticipated that use of "comic books" to explain risks, benefits, and alternatives to patients will increase. Likewise, a number of health care providers use videos so that the patient can participate in an interactive program as a part of obtaining informed consent.

From a legal perspective, it is always wise to document when videos are in use, document any upgrades of videos, and to ensure that the earlier versions of videos are saved and the dates of their use recorded. Often, when defense counsel is asked to meet with a surgeon on a case, more then 2 years have elapsed and the surgeon feels like lucky enough just to locate the chart, not to mention being able to find the exact video tape the patient viewed as part of the informed consent process.

The consent form itself is a document that does not reach the patient's hand until the surgeon has met with the patient, left the room, and instructed the nurse to get the consent form signed. It is highly valuable to have the consent form executed on the initial consultation visit if possible. It is preferred to have patients take a copy of the consent form home to review in case they have any questions. The benefit of having the consent form go home and being executed early enhances the ability of defense counsel to shoot down any attempt by the plaintiff to indicate that they were rushed into signing the document.

Much of cosmetic surgery involves direct payment as opposed to third-party reimbursement. Recent trends indicate that it is preferable to not have the surgeon involved in the discussion of the cost of the procedure with the patient. Instead, it is preferred that the surgeon delegate to the business manager or surgical coordinator the task of discussing payment issues and fees with the patient.

After an initial consultation with the patient, prudent surgeons may decide to obtain additional dental or medical records on the patient. I have seen cases, however, in which records come in to a surgeon's office and get placed in a patient's chart without ever being read. Certainly, situations will dictate that records be requested, and after they are requested, the standard of care presumes that they will be read. Hence, if you ask for it, read it.

Preparation

Advances in radiographic studies propel arguments by plaintiff's counsel that preparation in every case requires a denta scan or CT scan. Although panorexs or cephalograms have been the main radiographic tools for preparation, attention should be focused by the surgeon on determining whether advanced studies are warranted in preparing for a case.

Preparing detailed tracings, undertaking computer morphing, and obtaining detailed measurements to document a treatment plan are ideal ways to approach a case in addition to baseline photographs. Attention should be directed to the safekeeping of these items. The inability to locate drawings, morphings, tracings, or preparation materials 2 or more years after a lawsuit is filed can make what would have been a defensible case virtually indefensible.

Documentation

Surgeons ask, "What is it that I should document?" The key pieces of information to document are the words of the patient. Surgeons should place exact patient comments or statements in quotations in the chart because most states have a "dead man" statute that will prohibit a surgeon from being able to testify as to what a patient told him or her if the patient subsequently dies and there is no person or document to corroborate the alleged statement made by the patient. In other words, a surgeon is not going to be permitted to testify about what a patient told him or her unless it was witnessed by office personnel or documented in the chart, or both.

As plaintiffs' attorneys work through their checklist of items to determine whether they are going to accept the case and proceed with filing suit against the surgeon, one of the items often looked for is whether the surgeon has documented that all of the patient's questions were answered (the patient tells the physician that they have no questions or the patient had questions and they have been answered). Good documentation may well avoid a lawsuit entirely or certainly avoid a claim for lack of informed consent.

Surgeons have increasingly improved the rate at which they return patient telephone calls on a daily basis. What has seemed to lag is a willingness to document the patient's call and a word or two with regard to complaints or symptoms. The advancement in technology has brought to the forefront the issue of whether surgeons should consider communicating with their patients through electronic mail (E-mail). Several advantages to E-mail are that it allows the surgeon to communicate with a larger number of patients in a shorter period of time and that the message is a recorded document of a conversation. The downside to E-mail is the concern centering on confidentiality and privacy and the possible interception of an electronically sent message. Although an in-depth discussion of the pros and cons of E-mail is beyond the scope of this article, there are five points that warrant consideration as a physician ponders this issue:

1. Have a policy in place to ensure that E-mail is answered daily as are telephone messages.
2. Only agree to send E-mail to established patients who have originated an E-mail message to you using their date of birth and time.
3. Print the E-mail message after you send it to the patient or store it in a specially created file through your E-mail server or related software.
4. Do not copy any "cc's" or use the "reply all" function in dealing with patient E-mail.
5. Finally, make sure that your E-mail has automatic text at the bottom indicating that if there is a problem, the patient should immediately go to the emergency room and make sure that the text of your E-mail is deemed to be confidential.

After patients are given instructions, they will inevitably have varying levels of compliance. Historically, surgeons have been reluctant to document noncompliance by a patient, but that fear has given way to the malpractice crisis that now looms. Accordingly, when an appointment has to be cancelled, it should be documented not only that it was a no-show but also who requested the change in the appointment or what the exact nature of the noncompliance was.

The dictated operative report provides a surgeon with an excellent opportunity to reinforce all of the many steps that went into performing the procedure. The procedure can be viewed as a one-act play having several different preludes including informed consent, planning, and actions taken on the date of surgery. A surgeon's routine practice should be to dictate the operative report prior to proceeding with the next case and to note the time of dictation on the operative report itself.

Surgeons routinely ask about late entries in the chart. Late entries are red flags that are looked for by the plaintiff's counsel. I have never seen a late entry assist in the exoneration of a surgeon. When you see the phrase "late entry" in any medical record, you should consider whether the note should, in effect, start off with words along the lines of "I am going to get sued, so I might as well make sure I cover my tail feathers."

Postoperative communication

Communication with the patient can take a number of different forms. One form that has been found to be very beneficial is calling the patient on the evening of surgery to find out how he or she is recovering. Some surgeons elect to delegate this function to their nursing staff and to have an elaborate note entered the patient's chart. Although both processes have benefits, it is preferable that physicians make the calls.

Complications

When complications such as infection, excessive pain, or parasthesia occur, documentation should quantify and qualify the complaints. For example, How long has this problem been going on? What is the expected duration? What is the effect on the patient's ability to carry out employment duties? Is there any impact on the patient's lifestyle? Patients who are engaged in commission sales will often allege that they were unable to earn a living given their inability to communicate face to face with customers. Detailed notes in a surgeon's records can help combat those complaints.

When complications arise, it is essential to refer the patient to a specialist. A number of authors have advocated that referrals for nerve-related injuries must take place within 90 days of the onset of the injury and in absence of significant improvement. Because patients may not be compliant, the 90-day window, which seems long at the outset, can close quickly. It is recommended that when a patient is to be referred to a neurosurgeon, the referral take place sooner rather than later so as to not slip through the cracks. It is further recommended that anytime a patient is referred to the specialist, the appointment be made with the specialist from the physician's office. This practice will prevent the patient falling through the cracks and significantly prevent an abandonment cause of action.

Written communication is always a favorite target of plaintiffs' counsel. Be cautious of the way in which letters to specialists or referring health care providers are prepared. Letters of this nature should stick to the facts, be concise, and convey either an introduction of the patient or a thank you for referring this patient. Any additional strategies, side comments, and the like can give rise to the plaintiff's counsel being handed an argument of bias cover-up or the implication of "I'm just sending this patient to one of my good friends so he will look out for me."

Patient refunds and releases

Sears department stores (recently acquired by Kmart) achieve success selling their line of Craftsman tools by boasting a lifetime money-back guarantee or replacement on each tool. The American expectation of perfection has transcended department stores into health care: "If it is not perfect, I want my money back."Surgeons performing cosmetic surgery may be confronted by patients who think that the results achieved are less than what was intended and, therefore, want a complete or partial refund.

The decision to offer or provide refunds in an effort to preserve a patient relationship and avoid bad word-of-mouth publicity has prompted some surgeons to offer refunds to patients. From a public relations standpoint, refunds are logical and can be of benefit in the long-term. From a risk management perspective, a refund that is not handled appropriately can operate to fund a patient lawsuit against the surgeon.

It is recommended that surgeons have a policy that no refund will be provided absent execution of a confidential settlement agreement and release. Surgeons generally have their attorneys draft a simple release to use when this issue arises. Most of the time, the only aspects of the release that require modification are the patient's name and the dollar amount being refunded. Accordingly, a surgeon should not have to incur legal fees with each refund.

You should consult your own counsel regarding the wording of a release and the statutory requirements in your state. Most states have a statute that enables a person to rescind execution of a contract (including a release) within a certain number of days.

Confidential Settlement Agreement and Full and Final Release

This Confidential Settlement Agreement and Full and Final Release (hereinafter referred to as the "Agreement") was entered into pursuant to your state Code § code number in your city and state, as of __________, 2004, by and between patient's name (hereinafter referred to as "Mr. or Ms. Patient") and the name of your practice (hereinafter referred to as "the Practice").

I. Recitals

1. _________ received professional services and medical care from the Practice relating to list the procedure and dates of treatment.
2. _________ has expressed concerns regarding satisfaction with the health care provided by agents of the Practice.
3. The parties desire to enter into this Agreement to provide _________ a refund in exchange for _________ releasing any and all claims against the Practice and its agents, on the terms and conditions set forth herein.
4. Therefore, it is agreed as follows:

II. Release

In exchange for valid consideration as set forth in section III below, _________ releases and forever discharges the Practice, its agents, employees, shareholders, directors, insurers, or any other entity that may be charged with the responsibility for the events surrounding the professional services rendered from any and all debts, claims, demands, damages, costs, deprivations of right, loss of services, disabilities, expenses, compensation, actions, causes of action, contribution, suits in equity, attorney's fees of whatever kind and whatever nature, whether arising under state or federal law, which are now known or may hereinafter be discovered, as may have arisen at any time prior to the date of this Agreement.

III. Payment

In exchange for the release given in section II above, the Practice agrees to pay ____________ after execution of this Agreement the sum of $________________ by check. Such payment does not constitute an admission of liability and liability is expressly denied.

IV. Reading of Agreement

____________ warrants that he/she has carefully read this Agreement and warrants that he/she understands the contents hereof and agrees thereto. It being understood between the parties that _________ has not relied on any representations, expressed or implied by the Practice, as to the meaning of the terms of this Agreement.

V. Entire Agreement

This instrument contains the entire Agreement between the parties and no other promises or inducements made between the parties that are not contained herein shall be valid and binding.

VI. Controlling law

This Agreement shall be construed and interpreted in accordance with your state's name law.

VII. Confidentiality

It is further understood and agreed by the parties that the terms and provisions of this Agreement are intended to be kept confidential and only disclosed when required to do so by a court of law or state or federal statute.

WITNESS THE FOLLOWING SIGNATURES:
[PATIENT'S NAME – BOLD/ALL CAPS]
__Patient______________________
STATE OF ____________)
) to-wit:
CITY/COUNTY OF ___________)
The foregoing instrument was acknowledged before me this _____ day of ___________, 2004, by _________________.
My commission expires: _________________

____
Notary Public

____
THE PRACTICE ADMINISTRATOR

Summary

Although there are many keys that can be triggered in an effort to avoid a malpractice case, the two most straightforward and basic ones involve better communication and an attempt to document much more thoroughly. Avoid the urge to crawl in a hole when confronted with complications or difficult patient situations. Telephone calls to patients and personal notes will do more to benefit your practice than anything.

"What I remember, Mr. Johnson, is that my surgeon called me daily for the first week after my surgery, just to check on me. Although I was in extreme pain and was suffering, it was comforting to know that someone cared about my well being."

ELSEVIER
SAUNDERS

Oral Maxillofacial Surg Clin N Am 17 (2005) 129–132

ORAL AND MAXILLOFACIAL SURGERY CLINICS of North America

Index

Note: Page numbers of article titles are in **boldface** type.

1042-3699/05/$ – see front matter
doi:10.1016/S1042-3699(04)00135-9

oralmaxsurgery.theclinics.com

Changing Your Address?

Make sure your subscription changes too! When you notify us of your new address, you can help make our job easier by including an exact copy of your Clinics label number with your old address (see illustration below.) This number identifies you to our computer system and will speed the processing of your address change. Please be sure this label number accompanies your old address and your corrected address—you can send an old Clinics label with your number on it or just copy it exactly and send it to the address listed below.

We appreciate your help in our attempt to give you continuous coverage. Thank you.

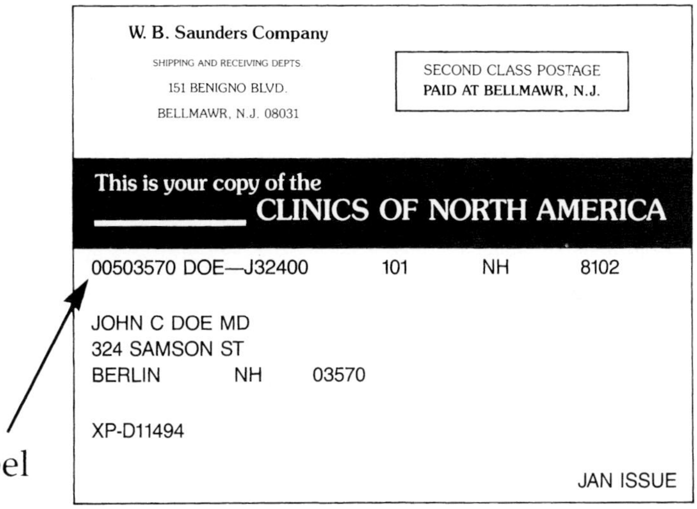
W. B. Saunders Company
SHIPPING AND RECEIVING DEPTS.
151 BENIGNO BLVD.
BELLMAWR, N.J. 08031

SECOND CLASS POSTAGE
PAID AT BELLMAWR, N.J.

This is your copy of the
__________ CLINICS OF NORTH AMERICA

00503570 DOE—J32400 101 NH 8102

JOHN C DOE MD
324 SAMSON ST
BERLIN NH 03570

XP-D11494

JAN ISSUE

Your Clinics Label Number

Copy it exactly or send your label along with your address to:
W.B. Saunders Company, Customer Service
Orlando, FL 32887-4800
Call Toll Free 1-800-654-2452

Please allow four to six weeks for delivery of new subscriptions and for processing address changes.